YOUTH
WITHIN

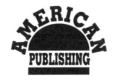

Additional copies of this book may be purchased directly from
the publisher. To order, please enclose $39.95 plus $4. postage
and handling. Send to:

Book Distribution Center
Post Office Box 15196
Montclair, CA 91763

Printed in the United States of America

0 9 8 7 6 5 4 3 2 1

TABLE OF CONTENTS

Introduction

I magine you are strolling in a park on a summer day and you are suddenly surprised to see an old childhood friend walking your way. You have not seen him in something like 45 years, but you still recognize him instantly. The first thing that strikes you is: *"My God! He certainly has aged extremely well! – if you can call that aging!"*

As you come closer together, you see the light of recognition in his eyes. He knows you too. It's been more than 40 years, but you grew up together as next door neighbors, and you never forget your best childhood friend.

As you come together and shake hands, you are embarrassed by your weak arthritic grip, while his hand feels firm and strong. You notice that his tanned forearm ripples with taut muscles beneath the skin. His eyes are clear and blue, and have that same devilish spark of fun-loving mischief you remember from your long lost days of youth. His hair is thick, full, and with only a hint of distin-guished gray at the temples. He stands erect with good posture — looks lean, poised and ready to play 18 holes of golf or a rigorous match of tennis.

You self-consciously suck in your flabby stomach, but doing so makes that twinge in your back jab with pain. Luckily, you're wearing a hat so your friend can't see the brown age spots on your balding pate. You gave up golf a long time ago because just swing-ing a club throws out your lower back every time, and you're out of wind after walking the first hole.

Still, it's great to see your old buddy, and it's grat-ifying to see that Father Time does not ravage every-one with equal fervor.

You exchange some initial words of surprise and affection. He's back in town visiting for a few days, then he's going back to his home on the West Coast, where he moved long ago.

Your friend spies a hot dog stand and asks if you want to get a snack, sit on a park bench, and catch up for a while. You say yes, but you have to skip the hot dog because it's been a long time since anything except boiled vegetables upset your stomach.

You settle for a cup of apple juice, while your friend gets a large hot dog with everything — hot mustard, relish, onions, a dab of ketchup, a garlic pickle to go with it — and a bubbling Coke. As he takes a first hearty bite, you notice a healthy looking row of white teeth — and they don't look false.

You shake your head in amazement. Time has been extremely kind to your old childhood friend — except the word "old" can only be applied to you in this case.

But the amazement is only beginning. You learn that your friend has not retired, as you did 12 years ago. In fact, he quit his job 10 years ago to strike out on his own and start a new business, which has grown steadily each year. This year he plans to expand overseas.

You are sad to learn that his wife of 38 years died in a car accident a number of years ago — but he has remarried and now has an eight year old son! With a wink and a nod, he tells you that he never thought sex would be so good at this point in his life! As for your sex life ... well.

Even though it's great to see your best buddy from the old neighborhood, an inner feeling of envy begins to boil over inside your mind! Something is truly wrong here! You feel cheated. You have grown old. Your friend has not! True, he doesn't look 18, but he also doesn't look a day over 40!

You finally give into your inner fuming (right after he mentions his plans for a hiking and camping vacation in the South American Andes next month).

You can't stand it anymore. You have to ask:

"Wait a minute, Bob! What's going on here? For me, a rigorous workout is a game of pool, and even that makes me breath heavy. You and I are the same age, but your going hiking in South America, raising an eight year old and expanding a new business! What on earth have you been eating!"

Bob chuckles and says: "You've got it exactly right, John, IT IS something I've been eating!"

Bob goes on to tell you that after his wife died 15 years ago, he was despondent, and the only thing that kept his mind off his great loss was keeping busy, and specifically, keeping his mind busy.

So he quit his job and went back to college. He majored in the toughest subject he thought he could handle — biochemistry. What he learned not only helped him overcome his grief, it changed his life forever.

You see, it was in college that he learned about the cutting edge of biomedical research, and that scientists studying the aging process were discovering amazing things about hormones.

Bob explains to you that specific hormones, which are produced naturally by our bodies, begin to stop their internal production as we grow older. A hormone, by the way, is a complex natural chemical of the body, produced by organs and glands. They regulate bodily functions of all kinds, everything from growth rate and sleeping patterns to sex drive and the aging process itself.

Bob studied biochemistry, and specifically hormones, for nearly eight years until he achieved a doctorate degree in biology, with an emphasis on biochemistry. Using the knowledge he gained, Bob convinced his doctor to prescribe a certain set of hormones which he could take in pill form on a daily basis, much like vitamins. It is this hormone therapy which Bob credits with not only the slowing of his aging process, but the reversal of many of the losses his body had given over to his "old age."

And here's what really stuns you: Bob says he fully expects to live to age 120 or 130! Furthermore, those latter years will not be the agonizing slow death of a withered, gnarled man slouching in a wheelchair, toothlessly gumming oatmeal or blended bananas, waiting for death day by day. No, those years will be vigorous and active right up to the end!

At first you don't believe him, but then you take another look at Bob and see the proof of it right in front of you. You and Bob are the same age, but he looks 25 years younger! That's a fact! Intrigued, you beg Bob for a few more details.

He gives them to you:

Ten years ago, Bob was floating in the same kind of leaky boat as you are in now, sinking a little bit each day. Just a walk across the street made him huff and puff. Arthritic joints made each movement a symphony of pain. His body was flabby, losing muscle tone. But his mind was still sharp, still young "inside." In fact, it was his eager brain that pulled him through the rigors of university-level study in a scientific field.

Taking hold of his new knowledge, Bob says he asked his doctors to examine his blood and to look specifically for the levels of a number of key hormones. Sure enough, many of them appeared to be in extremely low supply. It quickly became obvious why his body was aging and losing ground.

Most of the levels were at drastically lower levels than that of a 29 year-old man. That means that Bob's ship was not only leaking, but sinking faster with each lapping wave of time that slapped up against him, dragging him toward an inevitable "burial at sea" in just a few years.

But his doctors tossed him a lifesaver. They prescribed a series of hormones, specifically to counter the depleted levels as indicated by his blood work. The results were spectacular. Within eight months, his aches and pains were gone. He felt more energetic. Because he was able to move around more, he lost weight, and saw muscle tone returning. The spring was back in his step.

Everything about him changed. His skin went from sallow to vibrant, and even wrinkles smoothed out over the top of newly toned muscles beneath. His sex drive returned with a vengeance! He started noticing beautiful women again, something he hardly ever thought about during the past few years. It wasn't long before he started dating again, and in two years, he eventually married a woman 30 years younger than himself.

Their honeymoon was exciting, to say the least!

A Revolution is Taking Place

Bob's story sounds like something out of a science fiction novel, but every day, real science is turning science fiction into science reality. Biologists have unlocked the secrets of cloning, and they are mapping and manipulating the very building blocks of life itself — DNA. They are also learning things about certain body chemicals, including hormones, which are giving all human beings more options in battling disease and the aging of the body.

Certain precepts that have been true for all the ages are beginning to topple one by one. "Everyone is old at age 60, 70 or 80." It seems more likely now that age 75 should be considered "middle age." When a person hits 100, they may still have their best "golden years" ahead of them.

This youth renewal revolution is not being driven by a batch of flaky, alternative medicine hippy kooks who are concocting home-brewed fountain-of-youth formulas out of roots and herbs. Rather, it is the result of cutting edge research being conducted by some of the most prestigious medical facilities in the world, including Harvard University, MIT, the University of Minnesota Medical School, Stanford University and Johns Hopkins University.

A Hormone Primer

Before we continue our discussion, it will be very helpful at this point to provide the reader with a brief overview of just what hormones are and how essential they are in the very make-up of life itself.

Hormones are a tool used by nature in all her biological creations, even plants. Hormones regulate the fundamental processes of each creature, including plants, or that which creepeth or walks. Hormones control growth, metabolism, reproduction, and the functioning of various organs.

In higher organisms, hormones are secreted directly into the bloodstream by the endocrine glands. When everything is working well, and especially when animals and people are in a state of youth, a kind of dynamic equilibrium is maintained among the hormones, and they are able to perform their functions in surprisingly tiny amounts. The presence of hormones in all parts of the bloodstream create an effect which, although slower than that of a nervous reaction, is most often sustained over a longer period of time.

Hormones are produced mainly by the pituitary gland; the thyroid gland; the parathyroid gland; the adrenal, or suprarenal, gland; the pancreas; the gonads, or reproductive glands; the placenta and, under certain conditions, the mucous membrane of the small intestine.

The pituitary gland has three parts: the anterior lobe; the intermediate lobe, which is generally thought to be nonfunctional; and the posterior lobe. The anterior lobe is considered the master gland of the endocrine system. It controls the growth of the skeleton, regulates the function of the thyroid, affects the action of the gonads and the adrenals, produces substances that interact with those excreted by the pancreas, and may influence the parathyroids. It also secretes the hormone prolactin except when inhibited by the progesterone secreted by the placenta; prolactin stimulates the formation of milk in mature mammary glands. The anterior lobe also secretes the hormone intermedin, which stimulates the functioning of pigment cells. Hormones produced or stored in the posterior lobe increase blood pressure, prevent excessive secretion of urine (pressor-antidiuretic factor), and stimulate contraction in uterine muscle (oxytocic factor). Several of the pituitary hormones are opposed in effect to other hormones, as, for example, the diabetogenic effect that inhibits the performance of insulin.

The hormone of the thyroid gland stimulates general metabolism. It also increases the sensitivity of various organs, especially the central nervous system, and has a pronounced effect on the rate of metamorphosis, that is, the change from infantile to adult form. The secretion of the thyroid hormone is controlled primarily by the anterior lobe of the pituitary but is also affected by the hormones of the ovaries and, in turn, affects the development and function of the ovaries.

The hormone of the parathyroid glands controls the concentration of calcium and phosphate in the blood. The pancreas secretes at least two hormones, insulin and glucagon, which regulate metabolism of carbohydrates in the body. Insulin, which is a protein, was synthesized by American scientists in 1965, and glucagon was synthesized by German researchers in 1968.

The adrenal glands are divided into two parts, an outer cortex and an inner medulla. Extracts of the cortex contain hormones that control the concentration of salts and water in the body fluids and are essential for the maintenance of life in an individual. The cortical hormones are also necessary for the formation of sugar from proteins and its storage in the liver and for maintenance of resistance to physical, emotional, and toxic stresses. The cortex also secretes hormones that affect secondary sexual characteristics. The medulla, which is functionally and embryologically independent of the cortex, produces adrenaline, or epinephrine, which increases blood sugar and acts to stimulate the circulatory system and the sympathetic nervous system, and the related hormone noradrenaline.

The gonads, under the influence of the anterior lobe of the pituitary, produce hormones controlling sexual development and the various processes of reproduction. The hormones of the testes control the development of the secondary sexual characteristics of the male. The hormones of the ovaries are produced primarily in the ovarian follicles. These hormones, called estrogens, are produced by the granulosa cells, and include estradiol, the most important, and esterone, which is related chemically to estradiol and is similar in action but much less potent.

Estrogenic hormones interact with those of the anterior lobe of the pituitary to control the cycle of ovulation. During this cycle the corpus luteum is produced, which in turn secretes progesterone, and thus controls the cycle of menstruation.

Progesterone is also formed in large amounts by the placenta during gestation; together with the estrogens, it causes development of the mammary glands and, at the same time, instructs the hypothalamus to inhibit the secretion of prolactin by the pituitary. Various progesterone-like hormones are now used as oral contraceptives to inhibit ovulation and conception. The placenta also secretes a hormone, similar to one produced by the pituitary and called chorionic gonadotropin, which inhibits ovulation. This hormone is present in the blood in substantial quantities and is excreted readily by the kidneys; it is the basis of some tests for pregnancy.

A special group of hormones is secreted by the mucous membrane of the small intestines at a certain stage of digestion. They act to coordinate digestive activities, controlling the motility of the pylorus, duodenum, gallbladder, and bile duct. They also stimulate formation of the digestive juices of the small intestines, of liver bile, and of the internal and external secretion of the pancreas. The hormone gastrin is produced by one part of the lining of the stomach and is released into the blood by nerve impulses that are initiated by tasting food or by the presence of food in the stomach. In the stomach, gastrin stimulates the secretion of pepsin – a protein-splitting enzyme – and hydrochloric acid, and stimulates contractions of the stomach wall. Gastrin stimulates secretion of digestive enzymes and insulin by the pancreas, and secretion of bile by the liver.

Deficiency or excess of any one of the hormones upsets the chemical equilibrium that is essential to health, normal growth, and, in extreme cases, life.

The method of treating diseases arising from endocrine disturbances is called organotherapy; it involves the use of preparations of animal organs and synthetic products and has achieved marked, and at times spectacular, success.

When secreted into the bloodstream, hormones bond with specific plasma or carrier proteins that prevent them from degenerating prematurely and keep them from becoming immediately absorbed by the tissues they affect, called target tissues. Target tissues usually have receptor sites or cells that selectively trap and concentrate their respective hormone molecules, which are then held until the moment they are to react with target tissues.

Hormones are believed to affect target tissues in three basic ways. First, they regulate the permeability of the outer cell membrane and intracellular membranes. The hormone insulin is thus believed to relax the membranes of skeletal muscle cells, enabling them to transport glucose rapidly. Second, hormones modify intracellular enzymes.

Epinephrine, for example, coming from the adrenal medulla, enables the breakdown of glycogen into six-carbon sugars in liver and muscle cells by activating the membrane-bound enzyme adenyl cyclase. This process is mediated by "second messenger" moleculesónonhormone chemicals located in the target cells. When cell receptors bond with hormones from the bloodstream, they moderate the activity level of the second messengers, which either arouse or inhibit the target tissue.

The third way that hormones may affect target tissues is by changing the gene activity of the target cells. Either by directly entering the target cells, or more likely by acting indirectly through second messengers, hormones have been found to cause "puffs" in particular chromosomes, indicating that genes are actively involved in the synthesis of messenger ribonucleic acid (mRNA) molecules. The mRNA molecules, in turn, are translated into specific proteins that are necessary for such diverse hormonally produced processes as molting in insects or maintaining secondary sex characteristics in vertebrates.

Through recombinant DNA technology, or gene splicing, researchers have developed techniques for using genetically modified bacteria to produce insulin in quantity for diabetes patients. Similar methods are used to produce growth hormone, a substance in great demand especially for treating growth-deficient children. (By conventional methods, the growth hormone from 50 donated human pituitary glands is required for only one year's treatment.) Medical researchers have high hopes of using a plentiful bacterial synthesis to treat severe bleeding peptic ulcers and to reunite difficult bone fractures.

Scientists at these leading and mainstream laboratories are learning how hormones rise and fall in their production levels as people advance in years. Furthermore, they are learning which hormones play a key role in the major factors of human health and youth, and which are of lesser significance.

What's best, much of this research has already found its way outside of the laboratory, and is now available to doctors, who can apply them directly to helping the average person of the general public. Doctors are beginning to realize that they not only have new tools to battle the effects of aging — but that they can now have the added responsibility of treating aging as an abnormal disease!

Rather than just telling patients that they should "expect" their bodies to fall apart as they age, doctors can now take positive action to not only "hold" the body together, but return it to its youthful vigor. Helping people live to the "average" age of about 75 should no longer be the goal. Anyone who dies of "old age" at anything under 110 or 120 should be considered an individual that has been "cut down well before his or her time."

We already know that living to age 120 is possible. How?

Because a few fortunate individuals have already done so naturally, and without the aid of modern medicine! There are several hundred people around the world right now who are 100, 110; 120 years of age. If these people can live so long, theoretically, everyone with a healthy human body can do the same.

The answer for all of us seems to be hormones.

In this book, we are going to take a look at just that — super hormones that appear to play a key role in the aging process, and how replacing those hormones cannot only reverse the aging process, but help you regain lost ground and make you grow younger!

When discussing the aging of the body, hormone production, and such, many roads lead to a special gland in the body called the pineal gland. This tiny gland is located within the human brain at a position that places it right between your eyes. If you touch that midpoint space between your eyes with the tip of your index finger, you would be putting your finger on the location of your pineal gland. Interestingly, ancient mystics have long considered this area to be an important center of mystical power possessed by all human beings. In many traditions, it is called the "Third Eye."

In both Hindu and Buddhist Tantra traditions, it is said that the human body is actually an energy field made up of threads or filaments issuing from a central core — and tradition places that powerful core at the Third Eye, the location of the pineal gland.

Today, scientists are beginning to think the ancients may have been onto something. Up until only recently, the pineal gland has been considered a vestigial or "inactive" organ, its true purpose a mystery.

But now we know that the pineal produces the extremely important hormone called melatonin. As it turns out, melatonin is actually a transmitter of information from the pineal gland to the rest of the body. It also regulates a host of other important hormones.

Scientists have learned that just about all people produce large amounts of melatonin when they are babies and through childhood, but when they reach age 40 to 50, for some reason, melatonin production slows down dramatically. Because melatonin production declines, all the other important hormones it helps to regulate also suffer. At the point when melatonin production drops off, the body, as if on cue, begins to age more rapidly. Lose melatonin and lose your youth. It appears to be that simple.

Fortunately, something else may be just as simple: replace melatonin with supplements, and you slow the aging process, and even reverse some aspects of aging which has already taken place.

But wait a minute! Many of you may be thinking: It's dangerous to fool around with Mother Nature! Perhaps there is an extremely good reason for the pineal gland to reduce melatonin production at a certain age. After all, the body knows when to "turn on" the "puberty clock" when people reach their early teens. It knows when to "turn off" the growth hormone production, preventing people from becoming giants (except for those who have growth hormone malfunctions). Does it not follow, then, that a drastic reduction of melatonin at age 40 or 50 is just what the body needs to do?

Perhaps. But let's look at what good old Mother Nature is ultimately trying to accomplish. You see, nature by and large is not concerned with you as an individual. Rather, it is concerned with you as an entire species.

Nature cares about only one thing: that things keep going. Whether the individual members of a species live 100 years or two weeks is irrelevant —

as long as they continue to reproduce and exist. For example, there are some species of insects that have a total life span of just eight hours! In that eight hours, these tiny creatures do it all. They are born, quickly mature, find a mate, have sex, produce eggs which are fertilized and laid, insuring that the next generation will be born. They find time to eat something in between the maturing and mating. Then they die. They live a lifetime in eight hours. Their children will do it all over again.

Yet the species goes on. They exist. And even though each generation lives only 10 years, the species itself could live for millions! In the long-term view of Mother Nature, only the fact that the species continues it's cycle of life is important.

Indeed, all a human being really needs to do in terms of pure biology is to live long enough to reproduce, and make sure that its offspring are fed and nurtured to the point of being independent enough to mate and also reproduce ... and the process repeats itself off into infinity.

Mother Nature is simply not concerned with you as an individual. In fact, it is more likely that Mother Nature WANTS YOU TO DIE EARLY! Death is nature's way of making sure that the entire planet does not get crowded to the point of self destruction. The death rate must be fast enough to clear the way for each new generation.

From this point of view, it is logical for nature to build into each creature a "self-destruct" mechanism. In the case of human beings, that self-destruct mechanism appears to be melatonin — or more accurately, the drastic reduction of melatonin — leaving the body to age and die rapidly.

Yes, you may want to go on living as an individual. You have a unique mind. There is only one you. You want to know your grandchildren, to love them, to watch them develop their own special niche in the Universe. You want to have time to travel, sail, or idle away an afternoon by a beach or in a park. You want to create something that leaves your imprint, not simply the anonymous duty of reproduction. You want breathing room — to be able to contemplate the meaning of your life without death barking at your door just a few years after you retire.

But there has never been another species like Homo sapiens before. Perhaps when Mother Nature allowed us to come into existence, she had no idea what she was getting herself into.

That's because humans have an ability which no other species on earth has — self-reflective consciousness — the ability to know the self. As human beings, we comprehend time. No other animal does. Because we comprehend time, we know that our very existence has a limit. Combine our self-reflective consciousness of finite time with three things:

(1) our energetic desire to survive

(2) our consciousness of the fact that we are unique individuals and

(3) our advanced and growing ability to manipulate the building blocks of

Mother Nature, and it's only natural that we apply those tools toward increasing our own survival, not just as a species, but as individual human beings.

Still, some of the more philosophically inclined might say: "If Mother Nature has programmed us to die after a few dozen years, perhaps we should leave things that way."

This argument has some merit. After all, the world is already reaching dangerous levels of over-population. Each year, millions more are added to the planet, taxing the earth's resources. Soon, world population may lead to a crisis stage, meaning mass famine, wars, the outbreak of new diseases, not to mention to psychological discomfort of intense crowding.

On the other hand, we believe there is a different and perhaps more expanded way to view this situation.

Yes, nature built a self-destruct mechanism into the human body, but for some reason, it also allowed higher consciousness to develop — the kind of consciousness with the power to manipulate nature itself!

In other words, you could easily argue this: Mother Nature INTENDED for human beings to develop the ability to transcend ordinary biological determinism. The human ability to manipulate the building blocks of Mother Nature is, in fact, Mother

Nature's way of transcending itself. Mother Nature is in the process of creating something much more thrilling and miraculous than endlessly breeding, eating and dying biological organisms — it is creating meta-biological entities that will operate on an entirely new platform of creation, physical life and consciousness.

Indeed, it may be humankind's DUTY to transcend biology, and that means slowing the aging process, giving each human being more time to learn more, be more and travel to even greater heights of achievement and creation.

There is no problem human beings cannot confront and solve. Yes, more people living longer can lead to dangerous world overpopulation, but the same intelligence which is increasing the human life span is the same powerful force that can find solutions to overpopulation. It's thrilling to think about what the fantastic human mind will come up with — space travel, new methods of food production, or new forms of energy and engineering that will let 10 times the current world population live healthy, exciting, imaginative lives of more than 120 years for each and every person.

The starting place of all this is melatonin, which as we said, is an especially important hormone not only as it relates to the aging process, but in its function as the "master hormone," regulating the activity of several other highly significant hormones.

Most likely, you are familiar with or at least have heard of the next three. They are estrogen, also called the "female" hormone; testosterone, the "male" hormone; progesterone, also a "female" hormone produced in the ovary glands.

Now, several other hormones have been identified as major players in the youth renewal revolution. One that has been in the news a lot lately is popularly known as DHEA. This stands for the tongue twisting word: dehydroepiandrosterone. DHEA is now being sold on the shelves of every health food store in America since the FDA recently changed old federal regulations which did not permit this substance to be sold on the market. But now sales are brisk as word has spread that, among other things, DHEA is a powerful enhancer of the male sex drive. We'll discuss this and many other more specific aspects of DHEA later in this book.

Another master hormone is called pregnenalone. This powerful substance has been linked to improved memory and thinking, relief of arthritis and reduced mental fatigue. Pregnenalone keeps the brain functioning at peek activity. If you have a problem with pregnenalone, it manifests itself in a muddy mind, an inability to hold your attention on something or to concentrate, among other problems. Pregnenalone will be discussed in much more detail coming up in later pages.

Another important hormone is called simple human growth hormone. This substance is linked to building muscle, enhancing immune function, proper functioning of the heart, stress and kidney function. This hormone is perhaps the most controversial of the bunch, but also is a substance of extreme importance in the maintenance of an overall youthful body that can resist the ravages of aging. We'll take a close look at this important substance in greater detail in a coming chapter.

Yet another extremely significant master hormone is thyroid hormone. This provides the human body with a high level of energy, enhances immunity and regulates body temperature, among other functions. It's produced by the thyroid gland, hence it's name, but the actual stimulation for the thyroid gland to produce thyroid hormone begins in the brain. The brain produces what's simply called thyroid stimulating hormone, which goes ahead and does that.

The bottom line is, all these hormones work to make you young. When you are young, in your 20s and 30s, you have adequate levels of all of these hormones surging through your bloodstream and coursing through those parts of your body which use them to maintain peak performance. But as you reach your 40s and 50s, Mother Nature starts pulling the plug, and sure enough, you start to age.

But dwindling levels of these hormones does more than cause you to age. They also lower your resistance to disease. In the past 20 years the number of cancer cases has actually increased by more than 5 percent. This increase has taken place in the face of many tremendous advances in the treatment of cancer. How can this be? The answer lies in demographics. You see, the American population is aging rapidly. Today, with fewer births and better medicine to keep people alive longer, the segment of the population over the age of 65 is the fastest growing in the country. Cancer is largely a disease of old age. So with more old people, we have more cancer, even though we can treat cancer better, and even cure certain cases.

The significance of this is the observation that most common illnesses are diseases of old age. Yes, sometimes even children get cancer or arthritis, both those cases are aberrations from the norm. Most often, it is old age that lays people open to our most common diseases.

It is only recently that medical scientists have taken notice of this is a particular way. Rather than concentrating their efforts on curing a disease after it occurs, they began to look at how the disease could be prevented in the first place.

It is only common sense to conclude that there is something about youth itself that gives resistance to disease in most cases. What do young people have that old people do not? One of the clear answers is hormones at levels consistent with a youthful body.

It seems simple common sense then to artificially replenish those hormones which fade from our bodies with supplements as we age. There have already been thousands of cases in which doing so seems to work miracles. Rather than a steep decline from youthfulness into aging, those who replenish the master hormones we have mentioned above witness not a cessation of the aging process, but a much more gradual process that does not so much seem like aging, as a gentle transition into old age.

Yes, even with hormone therapy the body will eventually age, grow old and die. We are still a long way away from the deeper mysteries that sets the current limit of human life span potential at about 120 to 130 years. But if we have to grow old, the next best thing is to grow old much more slowly, and much more gracefully. Also, we can have a better quality of life in those later years, having bodies that are active and resilient to disease and constant fatigue for as long as possible.

Your Individual Hormone Program

Many people are making the mistake of running down to their health food store, buying bottles of melatonin and DHEA, and gulping them down in large quantities. This is probably not only dangerous, but may not accomplish the goal of reducing your bodies aging process.

Why not? The answer lies in the fact that each of us is an individual, both psychologically, and as it turns out, biologically. Have you ever noticed how some people in their 50s can look like they are in their 80s and ready for the retirement home, while other people in their 50s have an amazing level of youthfulness, both in appearance, and in what they are able to accomplish physically and mentally.

The reason is that everyone has a unique biological clock. Each person experiences hormone production at levels that vary greatly from one person to another. It's most likely a matter of genetics. True, many people are probably treating their bodies much better. Some people smoke three packs a day, eat fatty red meat every day, never exercise and have a lousy attitude about life. Without a doubt, these people cause themselves to age faster than people with no bad habits, who exercise regularly, and who maintain lean, low-fat diets.

Still, there are those extremely annoying people who seem able to break all the rules and get away with it. We all know people who are in their 80s and 90s who have smoked cigarettes or cigars all their lives. (Big cigar smoking George Burns who lived to age 100 comes to mind!) They drank heavily, messed around, slept around, had dangerous jobs, yet they defied all statistical convention.

On the other hand, there are those who live the lives of saints — vegetarians who meditate, have no stress, who are peaceful and loving, and who die of cancer at age 29!

Why does fate seem to be so fickle? Part of the answer lies in the individualized hormonal make-up of each person. Some people are simply genetically programmed to be strong and resilient, while others are weak and sickly.

Therefore, it doesn't make sense for everyone to gulp down DHEA or melatonin supplements in an indiscriminate fashion. It's a much better idea for each person to go their physicians, have a blood test performed and examine the levels of hormones as they exist in each person. Then, based on this read-out, the proper supplements can be administered to bring the body into optimum hormone balance.

Also, for those of you who take daily medications for pre-existing conditions, you MUST get a doctor's opinion on how taking hormone supplements will interact with your medications. Diabetics taking daily insulin, people with hypertension taking blood pressure pills, arthritics taking anti-inflammatory medicines — all of these and other folks must make sure that over-the-counter hormones such as DHEA and melatonin will not cause problems.

Once again, each person must tailor their hormone intake to a high degree. Furthermore, dosages of hormones may change from time to time as your body adjusts to it's altered body chemistry. Thus, each person with their doctor should continue to monitor their blood hormone levels, making adjustments when necessary, keeping an optimum balance.

Of course, many doctors are still leery of playing with the body's hormone balance. Very likely, your doctor will refuse to recommend that you alter your existing body chemistry with over-the-counter hormone supplements. It will be your decision as to whether you want to take your doctor's advice, or find another physician who is comfortable with such a practice.

However, as the idea of treating aging as a disease rather than a "normal process" gains advocates in the medical community, more and more doctors are going to routinely monitor the hormone levels of their patients, and perhaps recommend supplement programs to keep the body in youthful equilibrium.

Doing so can produce almost immediate benefits. Those who bring their hormones up to proper levels of quantity and balance find that their energy levels surge back almost miraculously. Their mood brightens, their sex drive returns, their minds clear, their muscle tone tightens while fat levels drop ... even the hair becomes more lustrous and full. Restored hormone levels also bring back the resistance to disease, preventing further damage and aging effects.

You might ask, if hormone therapy is such a great way to prevent the aging process and give the body greater resistance to disease, why are so many doctors unwilling to consider this course of action?

The answer is that just about all new and revolutionary medical advances have been met with a large amount of resistance by both the public and the medical community. It's all a matter of attitude. Although it is hard to believe today, many early physicians were actually fiercely opposed to the use of anesthetics for people who needed surgery or other painful procedures! They argued that it was "natural" for a patient to suffer pain, and that blocking the pain might be a bad thing for the body.

Today, many doctors have a similar resistance to countering the aging process. They say it is "natural" for the body to age, and taking steps to prevent aging may have drastic consequences. But by that logic, administering vaccines to babies so they do not develop polio is also interfering with nature. Administering artificial insulin to diabetics is also countering what nature has dealt to these unfortunate individuals. No doctor today would suggest doing nothing for a cancer patient or someone afflicted with arthritis. Yet, at the same time, they would say: "Just let people's bodies deteriorate with age. That's the natural way of things."

Doctors no longer have that option because new knowledge is making it possible for physicians to "heal" the body from aging. If doctors know that hormone depletion — hormone depletion which can be countered with modern medicine — is causing a body to weaken, sicken and die, they have an obligation to pick up the tools medical research has developed to "cure" premature aging.

Now that we have the ability to stop the aging clock, we must use that ability.

In this book, we'll talk much more about hormone therapy and how anyone can apply what modern science has learned so that anyone can benefit from the hormone revolution.

Beyond Hormone Therapy

While hormone therapy is new and exciting, it is not the last word on aging or preventing the aging process. The science of longevity has been gaining a lot of momentum in the past 20 years, and many other remarkable discoveries have been made about how and why the body ages, and what can be done to counter the aging process. In this book, we're going to take a long and fascinating look at a number of other major factors which can inhibit or slow the aging process and even reverse it in may cases.

In addition to the human body's naturally occurring hormones, there are many natural substances produced by Mother Nature outside the human body which seem to have a profound effect on aging. Among the most interesting are herbal and other agents from the plant kingdom that have now been proven to regenerate youthfulness on many fronts.

So in further chapters, we'll examine the very latest information on such exciting herbs as ginkgo biloba, an ancient species of tree which has survived more than 250 million years to continue thriving today.

Individual ginkgo trees live to be more than 1,000 years old. They are so hardy that a solitary ginkgo was the only tree to survive the atomic blast in Hiroshima, located very close to 'ground zero'! Ginkgos are planted as hardy shade trees in many places in the world, especially in cities, partly because they are so resistant to insects, bacteria, viruses, pollution and even old age.

Only in the last few years have modern scientists rediscovered what the ancient Chinese long believed about extracts and other products from the ginkgo tree — that it can pass on its incredible healing, survival and longevity properties to human beings.

In China, natural healers have used ginkgo nuts for thousands of years as a remedy for cancer, venereal disease, asthma, lung weakness, congestion, impaired hearing and to increase sexual energy and generally promote longevity. Today the ancient ginkgo has sparked renewed interest throughout the world because medical researchers have isolated chemical compounds from ginkgo that show startling effects in humans.

These compounds regulate blood flow to the brain, legs and other extremities and control levels of various neurotransmitters in the brain, thus helping to counteract memory loss, depression and lack of alertness which may develop in old age. These same compounds also block a substance called platelet activating factor (PAF) which, by over-stimulating the immune system, may lead to conditions such as asthma, toxic shock from bacterial poisons and perhaps even atherosclerosis and stroke.

Ailments Found to Benefit from Ginkgo:

- **Alertness, lack of**
- **Allergies**
- **Alzheimer's**
- **Asthma**
- **Balance Problems (vertigo)**
- **Blood Clotting**
- **Brain, Decreased Blood Flow**
- **Brain, Low Energy**
- **Depression**
- **Hearing Loss**
- **Hearing, Ringing in the Ears (Tinnitus)**
- **Heart Disease**
- **Impotence**
- **Intellectual Weakness**
- **Memory Loss**
- **Mental Confusion**

- **Parkinson's**
- **Senility**
- **Stroke**
- **Vision, Retina Damage**

Ginkgo is not the only rising star in the world of herbal anti-aging agents. Specific kinds of mushrooms, herbal teas and other extract agents are astounding modern scientists in their ability to stymie the aging process. We'll tell you all about it, and also tell you where you can find these inexpensive, safe and effective substances so that you can take advantage of them in your own life.

Other Factors Affecting Aging

Even if you balance the hormones of your body, take all the right herbs and vitamins, and eat all the right foods, none of it will do much good if you are living next door to a toxic waste dump that may be infiltrating your body with cancer causing industrial chemicals!

Indeed, what you protect your body from is as important as what you give it to keep it young and healthy.

Perhaps even more urgent is the fact that it is most often not something as dramatic as a toxic waste dump that robs your body of it's youth and exposes you to higher levels of disease and aging. You may be coming into frequent contact every day with environmental stressors which trigger faster aging without your knowledge.

Here are just a few examples:

- Too much direct sunshine
- Second hand smoke
- Exhaust from buses and automobiles
- Chemicals in your carpet, furniture, or wallpaper
- Common food additives you eat every day
- Common, popular foods that subtract years from your life
- Vitamin deficiencies
- Your geographic location
- The kind of car you drive
- Harmful soaps and deodorants
- Electromagnetic stressors
- Dangerous household appliances

... and many more. Every day, you may be coming into contact with youth-robbing and age accelerating agents, which you can easily avoid or remove to add decades to your life! We'll show you how to create a safe and sensible living environment for yourself based on common sense — and we're not talking about a life cowering inside a plastic, protective bubble! You can lead a normal, healthy life in the comfort of your own home without exposing yourself to environmental stressors that will land you in a nursing home before your time.

We'll show you how to stay young and healthy in a polluted world. We'll show how to avoid and detoxify.

No book on aging and youth renewal would be complete without a discussion of one of the greatest sources of youth known to humankind — regular, safe and practical exercise. While super hormones can keep your body balanced with its optimum body chemistry for youth, even proper hormone levels cannot overcome a slovenly lifestyle that has people sitting in front of a television for six hours per day eating greasy potato chips and swilling beer.

A body not exercised is a body abused, and sooner or later it will show the signs of neglect in the form of aging. You don't have to take up marathon running or join a health club for two hours a day of pumping iron. As little as 30 minutes of semi-rigorous exercise three to four times a week is all you need to stave of early old age.

Finally, Mind.

You know the old adage — you're as young as you feel. Sometimes the greatest truths lie behind the most hackneyed of cliches. Aging may literally be a state of mind. When it comes to aging, mind over matter may be the most powerful weapon we have in preventing the process of aging.

Most medical books on aging factors focus on the physiological factors or remedies that people can use to achieve longer life. They try to adjust and manipulate the physical body as if it were a machine that could be made to run efficiently and perfectly forever if only the right ingredients can be found and added to it in just the right amounts. That may even be the case and a large part of the total answer with the hormone manipulation we will spend many pages discussing in this book. But all the remedies and additives may be insignificant next to a few simple adjustments that you can make in your own mind.

Most doctors now acknowledge that millions of people "think themselves sick" every single day. Here's an astounding statistic: 2 out of 3 of all people in hospital beds today are not suffering from a genuine physical ailment, but from some kind of mental problem! Hard to believe, but true. All these people need is a simple switch of attitude — a genuine belief that they have the power to make themselves healthy, and they will be healthy.

This is not magic, or some kind of mystical voodoo — it's scientific fact. Your mind is indeed more powerful than your body. Your mind also has far more control over the rate at which you age than you ever imagined.

In fact, scientists studying experienced meditators have proved that human beings can actually adjust the biochemical make-up of their bodies through conscious direction of will. Those with a high level of mental control can adjust their heart rates at will, raise or lower their blood pressure — even increase or decrease the levels of the eight essential hormones we described in the first part of this introduction.

According to a study reported in the Journal of Behavioral Medicine, people who meditate on a regular basis have levels of age-related hormones that are comparable to those of non-meditators five to 10 years younger.

In the study, the level of DHEA of 423 meditators were compared to that of 1,252 healthy nonmeditators. The subjects were divided into groups according to their age, and meditators were compared to nonmeditators in the same age proximity.

Meditating females showed higher DHEA levels than nonmeditating women in every age group. Men under age 40 showed little variation, but after age 40, meditators began to show significantly higher levels of the youth hormone than nonmeditators. If 20 minutes of simple daily meditation can increase the natural level of DHEA in your body, that means that more than 20 other hormones which depend on and interact with DHEA will also get a tremendous boost.

Is gaining 25 to 30 years of increased life span worth 20 minutes a day of peaceful meditation? We think the answer is yes, especially when you consider that there are hundreds of studies which prove that meditation also increases happiness, promotes mental clarity, engenders higher spiritual awareness and improves the quality of life in many and far-reaching ways.

What good is living longer if you are not also going to be happy! What good is living longer is you cannot do the things you love to do, like travel, work on your golf swing, have a satisfying sex life, watch your grandchildren grow, create works of art, write a book, or just idle away hours watching waves lap up on the beach.

You can have it all. Let's begin our quest with the exciting world of hormone replacement therapy.

Chapter 1

The Amazing Fountain of Youth Hormone: DHEA

W e're going to start our discussion with a hormone called DHEA. You may already have heard of this substance, and seen many loud advertisements for it in newspapers, store windows, on the radio and TV.

Why has DHEA appeared so suddenly on the scene?

Primarily because the Food and Drug Administration (FDA) has recently lifted certain regulations which had banned the sale of this hormone without a prescription. The ban had a lot more to do with politics than medical science, but suffice it to say that government scientists have decided that DHEA at least can do no harm, if it produces so much good, as many doctors claim it can.

Scientists have known about and have been studying DHEA for the past 20 years, however, and the excitement in the medical community about this substance is high. **Here are some of the benefits scientists believe DHEA can provide for people age 40 and older:**

- **Restoration of energy**
- **Return of sex drive**
- **Improved memory**
- **Renewed resistance to disease**
- **Powerful stress reliever**
- **Cancer prevention**
- **Heart disease prevention**
- **Reduction of body fat**
- **Treatment for menopause**
- **Erases wrinkles, clears the skin**
- **Moisturizes the eyes**
- **Fights lupus**
- **Increases body's ability to heal**

These findings have already gone beyond studies with laboratory animals. Many people have already been taking DHEA supplements for as long as 10 years with nothing less than spectacular results. Here are some common reports of DHEA users:

"I thought I had forgotten what it was like to wake up in the morning and NOT feel like I had lead weights attached to my body. Since I began DHEA, I have the kind of energy I remember having when I was a teen-ager. I can work late into the evening, play tennis, and still get up the next day with no aches and pains, and feeling bright and awake.

— Shawn L. 55, accountant, taking DHEA for 6 months

"It seemed like only a few years ago that when I gained a few extra pounds, all I had to do was cut back on sweets for a few days and the weight would fall away. That changed. During the last few years if I diet for two weeks, I might lose a pound, but my energy level would be nonexistent, and I'd rather die than exercise. But since I began DHEA, I FEEL like exercising. My body seems to crave physical activity because I have so much extra energy to expend. Today, my weight has returned to my high school graduation level, and my body is firm and well-toned. It seems easy now to stay in shape."

— Helen, 47,
taking DHEA for 1 year

"It seems like I am starting on Life No. 2. My first life ended when I retired at age 68. I thought I would have perhaps another 8-10 years of sitting around playing cards and watching TV before going into a nursing home, or just dying from a heart attack in my bed. Nothing could be further from reality! I'm 75, and the last seven years of my life have been as full, active and exciting as my first years out of college. If I didn't know my age, I'd swear I'm 35! I'm starting a new business, not because I have to, but just for the fun of it. I have a lot of spare time for hiking and swimming, taking my wife on a third and fourth honeymoon, and helping my children with their busy lives. I see no reason why I won't be feeling great 15 or 20 years from now."

— Bob K.,
taking DHEA for 5 years

Such reports sound almost like science fiction, or fables of people who have discovered a fountain of youth. But the fact is, there are dozens of such actual case studies on file, compiled by research scientists and medical doctors who have seen the effects of aging completely reversed in elderly people who have begun regimens of DHEA supplements in their daily routines.

People of advanced age report the return of all the aspects we associate with feeling young — high energy, being clear headed, feeling ambitious, positive and forward looking, having powerful sex drives and being just plain healthy. Furthermore, the very common aches and pains which torment and slow many aging people loosen their grip and very often disappear completely.

The heart beat strengthens and stabilizes. The lungs go from raspy to clear. Sensitive and queasy stomachs, bowels and kidneys stop complaining about 80 percent of the foods which seem to bother most elderly people.

- **All this from a simple supplement that anyone can buy in any health food store?**
- **Is it possible?**
- **Just what is this hormone that scientists are calling the closest thing ever to a genuine Fountain of Youth?**

DHEA is short for the 25-cent word: **dehydroepiandrosterone**. It is a steroid produced naturally in the human body by the adrenal glands and by the brain.

While medical researchers have long known about the existence of DHEA, they have been puzzled by it. For the most part, they have considered it to be "useless." That's right. Because DHEA seemed to perform no real function in the body, medical researches concluded that DHEA was similar to the human appendix — a vestigial organ with no true function, and something the human body could easily live without. Yet, the body produces DHEA in large amounts. Why?

It was a French chemist who first found some answers. His name was Dr. Etienne-Emile Baulieu, and he decided to take a closer look at DHEA. He was able to isolate it from other steroids in the human body, and he discovered it was actually part of another hormone, pregnenolone. DHEA also seemed to be an essential building block of testosterone and estrogen, the male and female hormones. Doctors have long understood the importance of both these hormones.

Testosterone is what gives males their sex drives and is what makes males muscular and virile. Males lacking in testosterone experience obesity, lack of muscle tension and flagging sex drives, among other problems. Testosterone seems to be the primary substance which makes men what they are: generally more aggressive than females, deeper voices, larger, stronger, generally more sexually oriented. In a similar fashion, estrogen makes females what they are — softer, generally more passive and nurturing, higher voices and so on.

Interestingly, those people who wish to change their sexual orientation can do so by taking the appropriate hormone. Men who take high doses of estrogen can lose muscle tone, grow breasts, take on a more female figure, lose facial hair, shrink their penis size and generally become more feminine. The opposite is true for females who take testosterone. They can gain muscle mass, grow facial hair, deepen their voice and become more male.

But DHEA in and of itself does none of this. Rather, it is a building block of testosterone and estrogen, but by itself it seems a mere "inactive ingredient."

Many scientists were convinced, however, that the body would not be manufacturing such large amount of DHEA if is did not serve some important purpose. Perhaps more significantly, medical researchers began to realize that a body with very low levels of DHEA was a body that was old and deteriorating with age. It was clear that young people had a lot of DHEA and that old people had very little. In fact, a pre-born baby has extremely large amounts of DHEA, and DHEA, in fact, aids in the ease of the birthing process.

At the opposite end of life, when a person is near death, DHEA levels are almost nonexistent. A body depleted of DHEA is a body that is old and corrupted by age. It is significant to note that it is not the number of years a body has lived that is the best judgment of what shape it is in. Rather, it is the DHEA level which tells the true story. Some people seem able to stay youthful at age 75. It's no accident that these people naturally have high levels of DHEA.

DHEA levels tend to rise in the human body until the age of 20. At that point, it begins to decline by about 2 percent per year. At that rate, most people begin to feel a definite loss of youthful vigor by age 40, 45 or 50. As we said, there are exceptions. Some lucky people are naturally endowed with DHEA levels that remain high, but those people are very much the exception. If most people make it to age 90, they have less than 5 percent of the DHEA level they had at age 20. In other words — they are old!

Not only did scientists observe that high DHEA levels were synonymous with youth, they also noticed that high DHEA levels meant less disease, especially those kinds of diseases associated with old age, namely, cancer, arthritis and senility. Also, experiments on lab rats infected with cancer showed that injecting them with DHEA helped them fight off and shrink tumors with remarkable efficiency.

Because of these fascinating and promising results with lab animals, many medical researchers started performing human trials of DHEA. Nearly a dozen prestigious medical research facilities, including Harvard University, Johns Hopkins, Stanford and many others, administered DHEA to dozens of volunteers.

Research showed that DHEA was far from a "junk hormone." Those taking DHEA saw improved memory, renewed levels of energy, heart problems disappeared, obesity gave way to strong muscle tone, fatigue disappeared, mental clarity returned, strength and stamina increased — all the attributes of youth came back in force.

It will be helpful to take a closer look at each positive attribute provided by DHEA one at a time, and in greater detail, so that you can better understand the potential of this fascinating natural hormone.

Energy

A body that is not energetic may be young, but it will not feel young. For most people 40 is definitely not "old," at least not in terms of numbers. But if you are 40 and you just have no "get-up-and-go" you might just as well be 75. To be young, you must have the natural, inner energy that makes it easy for tackling any activity or participating in any sport you desire.

It seems that DHEA is an excellent solution to people who seem to have extremely low levels of energy. Doctors throughout the United States have already prescribed DHEA millions of times for elderly people with low energy, and the results have been exciting.

Donna L. is a woman in her mid-60s whose passion is her small hobby farm. Specifically, Donna loves mowing grass, trimming trees, landscaping, gardening, pushing around wheelbarrows filled with mulch and compost, building stone terraces and tilling soil. A lot of it is hot, heavy work, but as a child she was raised on a farm, and working with the land gives her a kind of satisfaction she can't get in any other way.

But little by little, "Father Time" began to catch up with her. As she reached age 67, 68 and 69, it seemed her ability to do all the tasks she wanted dwindled rapidly with each passing year. Every year her back would hurt a little more from bouncing along on her rising lawn mower. Bending over to rake or hoe her garden became a minor torment. Lifting heavy branches or the wheelbarrow were just jobs she could no longer do. Bouts of painful arthritis swelled her fingers, wrists and ankles, making each movement a symphony of pain.

Also, Donna just tired out easily. Only a few years ago she could putter around her farm for 8-10 hours, barely noticing she had not taken hardly a single break, other than a quick bite for dinner.

Visiting her doctor for her annual check-up, Donna's physician found nothing particularly wrong with her other than "old age." Donna complained about her energy level. Her doctor ran a blood test and found that her level of DHEA was low. He asked her if she would like to try DHEA supplements. Leery at first of taking any "drug", Donna asked if there would be any dangers or side effects to taking a hormone supplement. Assuring her that it was safe and that she could simply stop taking them anytime she felt uncomfortable, the doctor gave her dosage directions and sent her on her way.

After two weeks of taking a daily DHEA pill, Donna hadn't noticed much difference. A month later, she thought she still felt no different — except she began to notice that she was working longer, doing more, lifting more — and not taking as many breaks! Suddenly one morning she woke up, feeling not a single painful joint and feeling energized. She got up bright and early, ate a large breakfast of eggs, fruit and fresh-baked bread and went out to mow ten acres of prairie grass. She worked straight through some 5 hours to lunch and found that she had worked up a hearty appetite. After a delicious meal of homemade cold tomato soup and cold slices of beef with baked bread, she headed back out for a long afternoon of flower gardening and tree trimming.

At age 70, DHEA had given Donna her life back! She had almost given up hope of ever being "herself" again. But that's what DHEA did for her. It gave her the ability to be the person she wanted to be, the person she truly was. DHEA had given her the ability to live life as she envisioned her life to be. Just because she was 70 didn't mean that she had to sit in the shade sucking on a glass of weak lemonade through a straw, while a hired hand worked her precious flowers for her and a teenager got the lawn mowing done. For Donna, mowing the lawn was not a chore, but a truly rewarding retirement activity — and it was also just that — ACTIVE!

Of course, the primary problem with most so-called alternative health care treatments is that most of them base their claims on what is known as anecdotal evidence. This simply means that individual success stories are examined, while those cases where the treatment failed are ignored. Many so-called "miracle" cancer cures, such as the recent flaxseed oil flap or even the much vaunted Essiac herbal concoction are examples of natural remedies which gain all their purported evidence purely from anecdotal case studies. They zero in on those cases where people seem to recover almost miraculously after a week of taking a tablespoon a day of flaxseed oil or downing a few cups of herbal tea. The problem is that there is no proven connection between the remedy and the purported cure. Many other reasons can account for what takes place in these cases. In many cases, a person may have been misdiagnosed with cancer in the first place, a not uncommon occurrence. Or, some genuine cases of cancer do disappear spontaneously and without explanation. Doctors call this spontaneous remission and are baffled by it for the most part. Still, this does not mean the fold remedy worked. It simple means the cancer went away for some reason.

Finally, there is the well-documented placebo effect. A placebo is a neutral substance which produces no action on disease or the human body, such as a sugar pill, while the person receiving it is told that what they are getting is a powerful medicine. Sometimes the result is a cure. Although scientists do not know why, they know the body can be "tricked" into healing itself in this way, probably through deep, hidden and internal natural healing abilities which are built into the human body, but unknown to us on a conscious level.

But for a treatment to meet the rigors of true scientific respectability, it must perform with true statistical value. That means not basing results on anecdotal information which looks only at success stories — as in the case of Donna L. It also must rule out spontaneous recovery and the placebo effect.

The "acid test" of medical research on any medical product or treatment method is hard-nosed statistical studies, using what are called double-blind test cases and painful objectivity. The researchers must not be swayed by their hopes and expectation for the results they want to achieve. They must accurately observe results as they play out and respect those results.

These kinds of objective and statistically rigorous studies take time, sometimes years or even decades, and they also must be able to be duplicated by independent researchers with no connection to each other.

Fortunately, DHEA seems to be checking out under all these standards of proper scientific objectivity. In a recent study performed at the University of San Diego, one group of people were given DHEA, and another group were given what they WERE TOLD was DHEA, but was in fact only capsules containing sugar. The results were that the people getting the true DHEA saw tremendous transformation in their state of health. Their energy levels rose dramatically, they began to sleep better, wake up earlier and clear-headed, and within weeks began to gain muscle tone and lose body fat.

Some of those people who received the false DHEA reported improvements in energy and general well-being, but none demonstrated actual weight loss, clearing skin, loss of aches and pains, and so on. Some were made better by the placebo effect, but by and large, they fell far short of the people who received real DHEA supplement capsules.

Another area of improvement was sex. Let's take a closer look at DHEA and the libido right now.

DHEA and Human Sexuality

For the vast majority of people, sexual activity and youth are nearly one and the same thing. Many people judge themselves to be "old" when they notice their interest in sex has dropped off to next to nothing.

Sex indeed does seem linked to youth, although the vast majority of people do stay sexually active well into their senior years. Still, just about all elderly people drop off in the frequency of their sexual activity to a great degree.

DHEA clearly seems to change all that. People who start themselves on a DHEA regimen quickly notice that sex is something they would very much like to do again, and do it more often.

DHEA seems to be more helpful for the sex drives of men than women, although women also report higher libidos, probably more because they feel more energetic in general.

By age 70, some 15 to 20 percent of all men are completely impotent. By comparison, under 5 percent of men age 40 are impotent. Men younger than 40 have only rare incidents of impotency, and in those cases, it is often the result of a specific disease, such as structural damage to the sexual organs themselves, or diseases such as diabetes, heart disease or high blood pressure.

Interestingly, in those impotent men age 70 or over, the most common denominator among all of them is low levels of DHEA. There seems to be no other good reason for their lack of sexual ability than pure lack of proper DHEA levels. When discussing sexuality many so called experts make the mistake of looking only to the sexual organs of the body for the problem. What they fail to realize, however, is that the most important sexual organ in the body is the brain! This is where feelings of sexuality begin, where they are processed and where they end. The penis or the vagina is merely the "tool" which send the appropriate signals to the brain for processing. More than anything, the human being is a psycho-logical animal, rather than a biological one.

The point is this: it is difficult for a man or a woman to feel sexual if every other aspect of their experiences are laden with pain, physical suffering and lack of energy. A person in pain and with zero energy is very likely a person who is depressed and losing interest in life. Such a person cannot get excit-ed about the prospect of sex.

Thus, DHEA may bring back the human sex drive primarily by bringing back the entire system — ener-gy, freedom from pain, mental clarity, and a general feeling of well-being and optimism.

Thinking and Memory

Everyone knows that old people have poor mem-ories and that senility is inevitable as the years add up. Once again, loss of mental clarity is yet another of those attributes which we just accept as a "natur-al" and unavoidable aspect of old age.

Science now knows that this is simply not true. Aging people DO NOT HAVE TO LOSE THEIR MINDS! There is no reason that a person of 100 cannot be just as mentally sharp as a college graduate of age 22. And a big factor in achieving this state is DHEA.

Several careful, well-conducted studies involved dozens of elderly people who were deemed senile, "confused" or with actual an diagnosis of Alzheimer's Disease. A supplement of DHEA was added to their diets or was included with the other daily medications they were taking. The result in many cases was a complete reversal in all symptoms of senility. Memory returned. The elderly subjects reported being able to "think clearly" for the first time in years. Some felt extremely relieved that they knew "who they were" again, and were overjoyed to rediscover that they had friends, family and grand-children they previously had trouble knowing as anything but strangers.

DHEA seems to have a powerful effect in the brain's ability to process information. It does so by stimulating the production of something called neu-rites. Neurites are the individual building blocks and the actual biomechanical structure of memory itself. When a person learns a new fact, or stores a memory, in a kind of plastic fashion, neurites are formed and "glued' together in a vast, interconnect-ing network which make up the structure of memory and human thought itself.

As it turns out, DHEA is a vital and indispensible substance the brain must have to build neurites and neurite networks. As a person grows older and his internal rate of DHEA begins to fall off, the brain is literally be confronted with shortages of the very raw material it needs to not only build new thoughts and memories, but to continue to support its existing network.

In one significant experiment, scientists extracted brain cells from mice and also developed a method to keep them alive and viable in glass dishes filled with nutrients which feed brain cells. Researchers discovered that when they added DHEA to these brain cells, they grew much more rigorously, and formed thicker and more numerous neurite connections. This is very strong evidence that DHEA is a fundamental and vital building block of brain matter.

DHEA produced similar positive results in live lab mice with brains still intact within their bodies. Mice injected with daily doses of DHEA performed mental tasks, such as finding their way through mazes and avoiding electrical shocks, with spectacularly higher levels of proficiency than those who did not receive DHEA. Also, mice who had their brains purposefully damaged by researchers showed much greater ability to overcome the results of that damage when they received daily regimens of DHEA. Finally, mice who were allowed to age naturally and who had great difficulty in performing mental tasks on par with their younger counterparts were given DHEA. After just days of DHEA therapy, they begin to match the performance of mice who were in their prime.

Do experiments on mice mean that the same results can be achieved in humans? Well, as we have already reported, the answer clearly seems to be yes. In study after study, elderly human patients with all manner of mental problems, from deep depression and senility to hardening of the arteries of the brain and Alzheimer's Disease responded positively to the administration of DHEA.

Please note that DHEA is not a cure for Alzheimer's Disease, also known as AD. AD is a confounding disease with no known cause and no known cure. DHEA does seem to lessen the severity of AD, however, by allowing the brain to grow back many of the damaged neurite connections lost to the effects of AD. On the other hand, DHEA may be able to prevent AD from developing in the first place if an individual replenishes dwindling DHEA levels as they grow older.

The Immune System

The body not only grows old through aging, but by outright damage as the result of diseases which attack the body and wreak havoc on all the structures and building blocks of the physical system itself.

Eileen K., a 55-year-old First grade school teacher for more than 30 years, found herself facing a growing problem. Being exposed to dozens of small children every day meant that she was coming into contact with a veritable jungle of cold and flu viruses. A school room is a prime breeding ground, and small children who frequently put their hand in their mouths or up their noses get colds often. Eileen found that in the last few years, her resistance to these plentiful germs was growing weaker as she grew older. She was getting at least one cold per month. No sooner did she recover from one bug than another one hit her.

Eileen loved her job. Teaching and interacting with beautiful little children was her life. Yet, the constant colds, sore throats, respiratory infections, swollen glands and runny noses were making her life a daily misery. She seriously began to consider taking an early retirement. Continued exposure to so many cold germs was wearing her down.

During the first 20 years of her teaching career, Eileen rarely contracted a cold. Her youthful body and immune system were able to fight off most cold bugs. But now as her body aged, it was open season for germs and they preyed on her at will.

Eileen when to her doctor for help. He asked her if she wanted to try DHEA. After taking a blood test, he noticed her DHEA levels were low, and he immediately suspected this was the problem behind her flagging immune system. Eileen agreed to DHEA therapy. "I have nothing to lose," she thought, "and everything to gain."

By the middle of that school year, Eileen's colds stopped ... cold! Little by little, she noticed that she began getting fewer colds, and when she did come down with something, it didn't last nearly as long and was not as severe. The DHEA that was now coursing through her blood stream was providing her with a powerful boost to her immune system. Now she could fight off colds like a woman of 22. Best of all, she didn't have to quit the job she loved.

On top of that, she found that she had more energy to keep up with the explosive energy level of dozens of six year olds. Once again, DHEA had given a person of advancing years her life back.

DHEA clearly seems to fortify the body against disease, both minor ailments like colds, and major diseases like heart disease, hypertension and cancer.

A strong immune system is a vital component of being youthful and feeling youthful. It's difficult to feel good and energetic if you are constantly ill with something. Furthermore, illnesses take their toll on the body, so sooner or later, whether you are currently suffering from a disease or not, you begin to feel less yourself — in other words, old.

How does DHEA boost the immune system and help the human body fight off disease?

Nature has provided the human body with a complex and elaborate system for fighting off the literally billions of tiny, microscopic invaders that want to enter your body, use it as a host to multiply their own kind, and basically go on living as long as they can.

You see, viruses and bacteria see human beings as "food." They also see the human being as shelter. All they have to do is crawl inside our nice, moist, warm bodies where they have plenty to eat and plenty of room to multiply.

When an invading agent comes into the human body, however, the body does not take it sitting down. Within your bodies are special cells, which are a special kind of white blood cell called a T cell. There are many different kinds of T cells.

A suppressor T cell helps your body tell the difference between a foreign cell and the body's own cells. Obviously this is important because the body does not want to attack it's own cells.

Another immune system soldier is called the "natural killer" cell, NK for short. This entity patrols the body for invading cells and kills them. Still other cells are called macrophages, follicular dendrite cell and B cells — all of which work to fend off and kill invading germs that want to use and attack our bodies.

What's interesting and amazing about our body's natural defense force of cells is that they are able to "learn" or recognize a specific kind of invader once they have dealt with it. After they fight off a particular kind of virus once, you most often become "immune" to that virus for the rest of your life, even if you are exposed to it again. That's because your body has seen this bug before, has figured out how to kill it quickly, and does so every time it encounters it again.

This explains how scientists were able to develop vaccines against all manner of deadly diseases, from flu to polio. By injecting the body with a weakened flu germ, for example, the body's immune system gets a look at what it will need to fight it off should it ever encounter this particular strain of bug. The vaccine itself is not strong enough to produce a full-blown case of the flu, yet it gives complete immunity in most cases.

The natural human immune system is actually far more complex than we will explain here, but suffice it to say that the system nature has given us to stay healthy is mind-boggling, if not miraculous.

Yet ... Mother Nature gives, and Mother Nature takes away. As we grow older, those hormones which fuel and give strength to our immune system began to decline, and with it, our immune system begins to run out of steam as well. Often, the immune system can "get confused" in old age and start attacking our own bodies. This is how diseases such as arthritis occur. For some reason, our system of killer cells begins to attack the cells which make up the fibrous cartilage in the joints, connecting muscle to bone. The result is painful swelling, a wearing out of the joint and eventual total break-down of the muscle-bone-cartilage system.

Scientists are coming to believe that old, ineffec-tive and confused immune systems are suffering from a lack of those special hormones that give the immune system power and keep it working against invaders the way it should, rather than not working at all, or against it's own body.

Some extremely important substances in all these processes are called cytokines, produced by immune system cells. Cytokines are actually the communica-tion system of the immune cells. It's how they "talk" to one another, and coordinate their efforts in killing off invaders. Cytokines also tell the immune cells when conditions are normal and the attacks can cease.

In people with immune deficiency diseases, the cytokines are malfunctioning. They are sending all the wrong signals to the body's defense cells. The result is that the immune cells may lay around and do nothing while the body is being ravaged by foreign invaders. Or, they may begin to mistake the body's own cells as the enemy and attack them. Or, after attacking an invading disease, they may fail to get the message to "shut off" and continue to hammer away at everything in sight, like an army without a commanding general to keep them in control and tell them when to stop fighting. Out of control immune cells are like an army who defeats the opposing field of soldiers, but then go on to kill all the innocent civilians, including women and children, in the dwelling in areas beyond the battlefield.

DHEA has been clearly shown to have the effect of correcting the malfunctioning of the cytokine communication system in animals. In study after study with mice who had their immune systems disabled by scientists, injection of daily doses of DHEA brought their immune systems back into full operating order. Old mice who lost their immune system powers through age were also rejuvenated in their ability to fight disease by DHEA.

Recently the studies have gone beyond tests on the immune system of animals, both observationally and with direct experiments. It's no accident that young people with naturally high levels of DHEA are more resistant to disease. Now experiments have shown that people with low levels of DHEA and who are having difficulties with recurrent illnesses, can re-establish resistance by taking in artificial sources of DHEA via supplements.

Stress

The famous endocrinologist Dr. Deepack Chopra tells of an experiment on rats designed to determine the effects of high stress on a biological system.

In this experiment, researchers toss rats into a tub of water. They must swim for their lives. They are unable to crawl out of the tank, even if they swim to the side. There only choice is to tread water or sink. The rats were allowed to thrash around in the water until they nearly drown and then are rescued. After giving them a chance to rest, they are tossed back in again for another go. This was done repeatedly, day after day.

After a few weeks of this horrible treatment (a heartless experiment to be sure, even for rats!) the rats were put to death and then autopsied. Researchers discovered that the repeated exposure to extreme stress had aged the rats rapidly. These rats had the bodies of rats five times their age. Their muscle tissue was tough and leathery. Their bones were thin. Some had suffered strokes. Others died of heart attacks before researchers could put them to death.

The conclusion: high amounts of daily stress causes a body to age rapidly. Stress is more than just a psychological event. When a human being is under the gun, the adrenal glands produce what are called corticosteroids, which are chemicals designed to help the body get through a tough situation. For example, if a primitive man was suddenly accosted by a bear or a lion, nature made sure he had a chance to escape by jazzing him up with an internal concoction of chemicals, including the powerful hormone adrenaline, that would supercharge him for a burst of energy to either run like the dickens, or fight like a wild animal himself.

Stress hormones, as they are called, have their purpose. They help human beings deal with difficult situations. These hormones raise the blood sugar level, speed up the heart, get the blood pumping faster, expand the lungs so they can take on more oxygen, and so on.

But these reactions are designed to be extremely temporary, and ideally, stress reactions should not occur every day, every other day, or even once a week. If a primitive man were chased by a lion every day, he would soon end up dead, or he'd probably just give up!

Yet, the same kind of daily stress is what millions of modern day people must suffer every day. You don't need to be chased by a hungry lion to have your body trigger a similar release of stress hormones through the system. If you make a mistake at work and your boss bawls you out, your body reacts by releasing internal stress chemicals. If you live in a dangerous inner-city neighborhood in which a mere walk down the street brings the constant pressure of getting mugged, you are just like that primitive man in fear of being jumped by a lion. Your body floods itself with protective stress hormones.

But it doesn't have to be something as dramatic as the fear of getting mugged or being fired. Just getting to work every day — the cruel call of the Monday morning alarm clock which wakes you when you would rather sleep, the hectic drive to work on the freeway, the pressure to perform and meet deadlines at work, the mountain of bills you are struggling to pay, the house mortgage you are trying to retire, your relationship with your spouse if it is not going well — as far as your body is concerned, all of these things are the equivalent of that attacking lion. In a very real sense, many of us are like those poor rats hopelessly trying to save themselves from drowning. Your body is injecting itself with a daily dose of adrenaline and corticosteroids as it attempts to cope with the every day challenges of life in the modern world.

The ultimate effect is that you grow old and wear out faster. You age. Additionally, stress hormones weaken your defenses against disease, both minor illnesses and major illnesses. People who are under a lot of daily stress get more colds, more headaches, sometimes even migraine headaches, and always seem to be getting injured more often. Stress also clearly leads to major problems, such as high blood pressure, heart disease, hardening of the arteries, stomach ulcers and even cancer.

Because environmental stresses translate into chemical stresses in your body, it only makes sense, then, to take one of two actions, or both. First, you might remove the environmental stress. You might quit your job, sell your house, and join a Zen monastery, or take a long, winding cross-county hike across America.

For most people, however, simply quitting every-thing and walking away from their lives is impossi-ble. What about the kids? What about your house payments? Who'll take care of the dog and cats? What about your job and work, and what they have meant to you, even though it has been stressful?

Rather than running for the mountains, a second answer is to go straight to the biological problem itself. Wouldn't it be great if you could take in a mag-ical substance that would counteract stress hor-mones, neutralizing their effect, yet leaving you with the mental and physical ability to easily cope with your problems, meet your challenges — and feel great while you are doing it? Imagine simply not being affected by stress. Imagine not losing your cool, or getting hot and bothered by the daily grind, even when things are really bearing down on you.

Is there such a magical substance which can neu-tralize stress and help you cope with the hustle of daily life with a calm mind and confident manner? Yes — that substance seems to be DHEA!

We told you about the stress study with rats. As it happens, another group of researchers performed similar stress tests on both rats and mice but this time injected them with daily doses of DHEA. The results were again remarkable. The rats were able to endure their daily ordeals without the concomitant signs of physical aging displayed by those rats who were not given DHEA. In another experiment, a set of rats were injected with a substance called dexamethasone, a hormone that is very similar to natural hormones produced by the body during high times of stress. Most of the rats (again a cruel experiment, even for rats!) died within minutes or hours of strokes and heart attacks. They also became markedly agitated.

Next, a second group of rats were fortified with injections of DHEA. These rats were also given injections of dexamethasone. The result? No strokes, heart attacks or raised blood pressure. DHEA truly seemed to have neutralized the stress hormones in these animals.

Although much more thorough studies need to be done on the effects of DHEA and stress on human beings, there is already scads of anecdotal evidence being reported by people who are actually taking DHEA that it is a powerful counter measure against stress. Many high pressure doctors, lawyers, journalists and others have reported a much greater capacity to handle the daily stress of their jobs without "losing their cool" or experiencing that tell-tale feeling of having all the blood rise to their heads making it throb and eventually produce a migraine, hypertension, or just plain old agitation.

Preventing stress is important because many common illnesses develop as a result of stress. Doctors believe a whole catalog of diseases, especially hypertension, ulcers, arthritis, diabetes, heart disease, chronic migraine headaches, insomnia and many others are all stress induced or stress-related illnesses.

DHEA's possible ability to block stress hormones from forming in the human body may not only mean millions of people will have easier psychological burdens in their day-to-day lives, but less actual physical disease which further robs the body of youth and vitality.

So in addition to simply feeling better about coping with the daily stress of living, DHEA can also stop stress from breaking down the body and aging it before its time.

DHEA and Cancer

Studies that have been going on at Temple University in Philadelphia for some 20 years have been looking at a possible connection between DHEA and cancer, or more accurately, the strong possibility that DHEA prevents cancer.

As we said earlier, cancer is primarily a disease of old age. A man of age 70 is more than 60 times more likely to develop cancer than a man in his 20s. As the body ages, it loses its ability to fight off diseases as we have seen. It also loses its resistance to one of nature's most deadly killers — cancer.

It stands to reason that if the human body could be kept from getting old, its chances of contracting cancer would diminish accordingly. If a 20-year-old man has only a tiny chance of getting cancer, can we give a 70-year-old man the same chance by matching the biochemical make-up of the younger man.

Cancer is actually an "inside job." By that we mean cancer involves not an invading foreign microbe or germ, but one of the body's own cells which has "gone bad." This cell begins to grow for its own sake rather than serving its normal function as a member of the family of cells which make up the human body. A cancer cell writes its own DNA patterns and starts a colony of its own kind, forming a tumor. This tumor begins to damage the organs it is attached to and also robs the rest of the body of the energy it needs to function properly.

Much cancer probably starts when a cell is negatively affected by an outside source, such as radiation, a toxic substance, cigarette smoke, or even too much sunlight. A cancer cell can also just "go bad" on its own due to a genetic flaw inherent in the cell's DNA.

Chemical Causes of Cancer

Chemical agents that cause cancer have been extensively studied by medical research scientists Some chemicals act as initiators. Only a single exposure is required, but cancer does not follow until after a long latent period and after exposure to another agent that acts as a promoter. Initiators produce irreversible changes in DNA. Promoters do not change DNA, but they do increase synthesis of DNA and stimulate expression of genes. They have no effect if given before the initiator, only if given after the initiator and given repeatedly over a period of time.

Tobacco smoke contains many chemical initiators and promoters. The promoter action of cigarettes is very important, and if smoking is stopped, the risk of lung cancer falls rapidly. Alcohol is an important promoter; chronic abuse greatly increases the risk of cancers known to be induced by other agents, such as lung cancer in smokers. Carcinogenic chemicals also produce chromosome breaks and translocations. See also Carcinogen.

Immune System Factors

The immune system appears to be able to recognize malignant cells and stimulate the production of cells able to destroy them. An important factor in the development of cancer may be a disease or other damaging event leading to a state of immune deficiency. Such states are a consequence of AIDS, inherited immune deficiency diseases, and the administration of immunosuppressive drugs.

Environmental Factors

It is estimated that about 80 percent of cancers may be caused by environmental factors. The best established cause is tobacco smoke, actively or passively inhaled, which is responsible for about 30 percent of all deaths from cancer in the U.S. Dietary factors may account for about 40 percent, but the causative relationship is not as clear, and the responsible constituents of the diet are not clearly defined. Obesity is a risk factor for a number of cancers, especially cancers of the breast, colon, uterus, and prostate. Dietary fat and low dietary fiber are associated with high incidence of colon cancer. Dietary fat and obesity, like alcohol, appear to act as promoters.

The Oncogene

The common component that unites these seemingly disparate mechanisms may be the oncogene. Oncogenic viruses may insert their genes at many loci in the animal genome. A viral oncogene that is inserted in connection with a cellular oncogene influences the expression of the oncogene and induces cancer. Radiation and carcinogenic chemicals produce DNA damage, mutations, and chromosome changes, and oncogenes are often located on the chromosome near the fragile site or breakpoint.

A malignancy appears to be the result of a series of mishaps beginning with an abnormal gene or a somatic mutation, probably more than one, followed by a promoting activity that stimulates the expression of one or more oncogenes, leading to the release of growth factors. Perhaps the earlier event leads to the loss of production of metabolites necessary for the normal differentiation of the cell. The stimulation of growth factors then causes the clone of undifferentiated cells to proliferate, and a defect in the immune system permits the abnormal cells to escape destruction by the normal surveillance mechanism.

Occurrence

More than 1 million new cases of cancer occur in the U.S. each year. It is the second leading cause of death in the nation, accounting for about 500,000 deaths annually, and is the leading cause of death from disease in children between the ages of 1 and 14. The incidence of cancer varies enormously among different geographic areas. The age-adjusted death rate from all cancers in males is 310.9 per 100,000 in Luxembourg (the highest) as compared to 37.5 in El Salvador (the lowest). For women it is 175.2 in Denmark and 48.7 in El Salvador. The figures for the U.S. are 216.6 per 100,000 men and 136.5 per 100,000 women. For particular cancers the difference between countries may be as high as 40-fold. Evidence from studies of populations that have migrated from one geographic area to another suggests that these variations are due to differences in life-style rather than ethnic origin. This is consistent with other evidence that most cancers are predominately related to environmental causes rather than heredity, although the two interact.

The cancers that cause the most deaths in the U.S. are lung cancer (first in each sex), colorectal cancer (second in both sexes combined), breast and uterine cancers in women, and prostate cancer in men. Together they account for more than 55 percent of all deaths from cancer. The most frequently occurring cancers are cancers of the skin, with over 500,000 cases per year, which, except for malignant melanoma, are not counted in the statistics.

Since 1949 cancer mortality in the U.S. has been higher among men than among women. The sex ratios of different cancers vary considerably. Cancer mortality is higher among blacks than whites for reasons that are not fully understood but are under intensive study.

Mother Nature is familiar with cancer, having encountered it billions of times over the centuries.

Because of this, it has given most human beings a natural defense system to fight off cancer. Some scientists are now coming to believe that DHEA may be one of nature's primary, natural anti-cancer mechanisms.

Studies show that DHEA may stop cancer almost as soon as it gets started. It does this with an enzyme in the human body called glucose-6-phosphate dehydrogenase, called G6PDH for short. This substance "alerts" cancer cells to come awake and start growing. If G6PDH could be stopped, even an existing cancer cell in the body could do little harm because it could not reproduce and begin ravaging and taking over the rest of the body. Studies indicate that DHEA may do just that — put a lid on G6PDH.

A Free Radical Scrubber

Later in this book we are going to tell you about foods and vitamins that are important in preventing both aging and cancer because they remove something from the body called "free radicals."

You might say that free radicals are oxygen molecules that have "gone bad." The human body uses oxygen to help metabolize energy. But some of those oxygen molecules are damaged in the process. Some individual oxygen molecules are stripped of one of their outer electrons, leaving them in an unstable condition. If you remember a bit of your high school chemistry, all molecules do not like to remain "incomplete" or out of balance. Damaged oxygen molecules are pulled toward other molecules in the body so they can bond with them, and thus stabilize themselves. But when a free radical oxygen molecule unites with an atom of the body it causes a tiny bit of damage, weakening that atom, which is a component of a larger cell. If there are enough free radicals floating around in the body the forced bonding begins to cause large-scale cellular damage.

During the last decade, this free radical action has been the focus of much intense interest by the medical community. It is still considered to be an important — if not THE — key in understanding the aging process, and in understanding why some cells develop into cancer cells.

Furthermore, scientists have been surprised that certain common substances have the effect of eliminating free radical atoms from the body, the four most common being vitamin C, Vitamin A, Vitamin E and beta-carotene. (There are others, but these seem to be the most powerful "free radical scrubbers".)

But while these excellent and healthy substances do a good job of cleaning up free radicals after they have been released into the body, it may be that DHEA is a superior agent against free radicals because it PREVENTS THEM FROM BEING FORMED IN THE FIRST PLACE! **DHEA may very well be the perfect antioxidant.**

Recently, physicians diagnosed an 87-year-old man, whom we'll call Max, with lung cancer. After several rounds of chemotherapy and radiation, little had been done to slow the spread of his disease. Yet, the elderly gentleman suffered greatly from the ravages of the treatment. He lost nearly 20 pounds. He was open to attack from all kinds of cold and other viruses because of the devastating effect the chemo had on his immune system. He had little appetite and was getting weaker by the day. He was in pain. His eyesight had grown dim and even his hearing had been reduced.

Although most think 87 is a very old age, Max had been extremely vigorous right up to the time doctors discovered his cancer six months ago. Up until that time, most would have mistaken him for 62. He was an avid hiker and hunter. He still worked part-time in a business of his own. He was dating a woman about 15 years his junior.

But just six months of conventional cancer treatment had changed all that with surprising rapidity. Now, he looked every day of his 87 years, and in fact, looked closer to 100. Max was ready to give up and simply die. And he had had it with chemotherapy and radiation. If that's what he has to go through to live, death would be a welcome release, he told his doctors.

Judging his case to be all but hopeless, Max's doctors asked him if he would like to try one last thing — a daily regimen of DHEA therapy. They told him that taking DHEA would not be a harsh treatment as was chemo and radiation. They also cautioned him not to get his hopes up because, to date, very little evidence had been gathered as to DHEA effectiveness against cancer, if it had any effect on cancer at all. Max readily agreed to both DHEA treatment, and to taking a battery of other antioxidant substances, including vitamin's C, E, A and beta carotene, among others. He had absolutely nothing to lose.

The results were remarkable. Within just two weeks, Max began to get his strength back. His lungs were no longer filling with cancerous fluid. The spread of his cancer seemed to have stopped cold and even recede. Shortly, Max felt like eating again, and with the return of his appetite, his old "die-hard" positive outlook came back. Within two months, Max was back doing the things he loved to do — hiking, hunting, spending time with his lady friend and running his small business.

Of course, the case of Max represents a statistic of one, and not an entire scientific study of thousands of cancer patients and DHEA treatment. Until that kind of data is obtained, it will be impossible to conclude that DHEA can actually stop and reverse cancer. Still, the growing anecdotal evidence is both exciting and promising. Also, because of the safety and lack of serious side effects of traditional cancer treatments, there is nothing to stop more doctors from trying DHEA on more cancer patients and growing the baseline of data available on cancer and DHEA.

DHEA — a New Class of Drug Treatment?

Just one class of drugs almost instantly added 20 to 30 years of life to the average human being. The first of that class of drugs was called penicillin, just one of many antibiotics that were to follow.

We take antibiotics for granted today, but just a few decades ago, millions of people died from infections of all kinds, many of which we would consider minor today. Step on a nail? Your dead! Get an infected tooth? It could kill you! Get bitten by a dog? It may very likely end your life! Drink some bad water? It may send you to your grave!

Today, if you step on a nail, you stop at a local clinic for a tetanus shot, and you forget about it. Infections? No problem! Medical science has a battery of antibiotics to counter thousands of germs Mother Nature serves up to us in our every day environment. Yes, it's true that thousands of people still succumb to infections every day, and that even our best antibiotics sometimes fail, but the net result of antibiotics has translated into years of added life expectancy for every human being on the planet with access to modern medicine.

The first antibiotic was developed in the 19th century by the French chemist Louis Pasteur, who discovered that certain saprophytic bacteria can kill anthrax germs. Then, in the year 1900 the German bacteriologist Rudolf von Emmerich developed a substance called pyocyanase, which can kill the germs of cholera and diphtheria in the test tube. It was not useful, however, in curing disease.

In the 1920s the British bacteriologist Sir Alexander Fleming, who later discovered penicillin, found a substance called lysozyme in many of the secretions of the body, such as tears and sweat, and in certain other plant and animal substances. Lysozyme has strong antimicrobial activity, but mainly against harmless bacteria.

Penicillin, the archetype of antibiotics, was discovered by accident in 1928 by Fleming, who showed its effectiveness in laboratory cultures against many disease-producing bacteria, such as those that cause gonorrhea and certain types of meningitis and bacteremia (blood poisoning); however, he performed no experiments on animals or humans. Penicillin was first used on humans by the British scientists Sir Howard Florey and Ernst Chain during the 1940-41 winter.

The first antibiotic to be used in the treatment of human diseases was tyrothricin (one of the purified forms of which was called gramicidin), isolated from certain soil bacteria by the American bacteriologist Rene' Dubos in 1939. This substance is too toxic for general use, but it is employed in the external treatment of certain infections. Other antibiotics produced by actinomycetes (filamentous and branching bacteria) occurring in soil have proved more successful. One of these, streptomycin, discovered in 1944 by the American microbiologist Selman Waksman and his associates, is effective against many diseases, including several in which penicillin is useless, especially tuberculosis.

Since then, such antibiotics as chloramphenicol, the tetracyclines, erythromycin, neomycin, nystatin, amphotericin, cephalosporins, and kanamycin have been developed and may be used in the treatment of infections caused by some bacteria, fungi, viruses, rickettsia, and other micro-organisms. In clinical treatment of infections, the causative organism must be identified and the antibiotics to which it is sensitive must be determined in order to select an antibi-

otic with the greatest probability of killing the infect-
ing organism.

Strains of bacteria have arisen that are resistant to
commonly used antibiotics; for example, gonorrhea-
causing bacteria that high doses of penicillin are not
able to destroy may transfer this resistance to other
bacteria by exchange of genetic structures called
plasmids. Some bacteria have become simultaneously resistant to two or more antibiotics by this mechanism. New antibiotics that circumvent this problem, such as the quinolones, are being developed.
The cephalosporins, for instance, kill many of the
same organisms that penicillin does, but they also
kill strains of those bacteria that have become resistant to penicillin. Often the resistant organisms arise
in hospitals, where antibiotics are used most often,
especially to prevent infections from surgery.

Another problem in hospitals is that many old and
very ill persons develop infections from organisms
that are not pathogenic in healthy persons, such as
the common intestinal bacterium Escherichia coli.
New antibiotics have been synthesized to combat
these organisms. Fungus infections have also
become more common with the increasing use of
chemotherapeutic agents to fight cancer, and more
effective antifungal drugs are being sought.

The search for new antibiotics continues in general, as researchers examine soil molds for possible
agents. Among those found in the 1980s, for example, are the monobactams, which may also prove
useful against hospital infections. Antibiotics are
found in other sources as well, such as the family of

magainins discovered (in the late 1980s) in frogs; although untested in humans as yet, they hold broad possibilities.

Another example of a class of drugs that has prevented untold millions of premature deaths are vaccines, which provide immunity to diseases.

Immunization is the process of rendering people immune to an infectious organism by inoculating them with a form of the organism that does not cause severe disease but does provoke formation of protective antibodies. The process has also been called vaccination, because the first instance of immunization was the use of vaccinia, or cowpox, virus to produce immunity to variola, or smallpox.

Vaccines are the most effective protection against most diseases caused by viruses and related organisms, because few antibiotics work against them. In Western countries vaccines are routinely used in the first years of life to produce immunity to diphtheria, tetanus, poliomyelitis, and whooping cough. See also Immune System.

A vaccine may contain organisms killed by exposure to heat or chemicals (the first polio vaccine, and one for typhoid fever); an inactivated form of a toxin, produced by the organism and called a toxoid (tetanus and diphtheria vaccines); or a live attenuated virus, one grown in such a way that it can no longer cause serious disease (the polio vaccine developed by Albert Sabin, and vaccines against measles and yellow fever).

The first modern use of immunization was by the British physician Edward Jenner in 1796, when he used cowpox inoculations to produce protection against smallpox. In 1885 the French scientist Louis Pasteur first used an attenuated rabies virus to protect against the natural infection, and in 1897 a vaccine against typhoid fever was developed in England.

The immunizing substance is usually introduced through a scrape in the skin, called inoculation, although the Sabin polio vaccine is taken orally. Protection lasts for varying periods: the plague vaccine for only six months; the yellow fever vaccine for ten years.

A population can be immunized in two ways. In one method, the vaccine is targeted to those most likely to get the disease. In the recent successful campaign to eradicate smallpox worldwide, a form of this strategy was used. Most diseases in Western countries, on the other hand, are controlled through the principle of herd immunity, in which it is held that the transmission of disease will be stopped when an extremely low probability exists that an infected person will come into contact with an unprotected individual. Not every person needs to be immunized, but protection levels of 90 percent must be reached for some diseases. In some instances a combined strategy is used. For rubella, or German measles, for example, public health workers aim at mass immunization of school-age children as well as of women of childbearing age.

Immunization remains one of the primary weapons in the fight against infectious disease. In

1977 the U.S. government earmarked $57 million to promote measles immunization; many states adopted the rule that children could not enter school without a certificate of measles immunization, and they also provided programs for those not immunized. The effort was so effective that the incidence of measles had dropped to record lows by the early 1980s; with cutbacks in funding, however, the incidence of the disease had risen significantly by the early 90s.

New vaccines are still being developed, such as a safer, less painful vaccine against rabies and vaccines against hepatitis B and pneumonia-causing bacteria. Third World diseases for which vaccines are being sought include cholera and parasitic infections such as malaria and trypanosomiasis. In addition to active immunization (stimulating antibody formation by introducing a form of the infectious organism), protection may also be provided by passive immunization (injecting serum containing antibodies, usually obtained from a person who has recently had the disease). The latter procedure is now seldom used, except in some cases of hepatitis.

Fifty years from now, historians may be looking back on the 1990s as the decade when another class of drugs with the stature of antibiotics and vaccines was added to life-saving and life-extending arsenal of modern medicine. Primary among those may be DHEA.

One of the primary ways that DHEA may allow millions of people to live beyond the average age of 75 or so is by preventing one of the top killers of all people today — heart disease. The American Heart Association says that if heart disease were eliminated today, the average human life expectancy could be immediately increased from 75 to 80 or 95.

In addition to extending life, a healthy heart adds quality to life. Many people struggle through the last 20 years of their lives with a weak heart, making them all but helpless to perform all but the simplest activities for themselves.

People with bad hearts get short of breath after just a walk across the living room. Any strenuous activity could result in death due to heart failure.

Today, many medical researchers think DHEA may be a key to preventing heart disease from developing in the first place, and stopping the progression of heart disease in those people who already have a problem.

(Please note: Smoking cigarettes is still the No. 1 cause of heart disease in the world today. Even without possible new treatments such as DHEA therapy, if people simply avoided tobacco products, a large majority of all heart problems would also disappear, and the average life expectancy of humans would be increased as well.)

To understand how people get heart disease and how DHEA may be able to prevent it, it will be helpful here to briefly explain how heart disease develops. As we said, heart disease kills more Americans than any other disease, even more than cancer. Heart problems arise from congenital defects, infections, narrowing of the coronary arteries, high blood pressure, or disturbances of heart rhythm.

Congenital heart defects include persistence of fetal connections between the arterial and venous circulations, such as the ductus arteriosus, a vessel normally connecting the pulmonary artery and the aorta only until birth.

Other problems involve the partition separating the four cardiac cavities and the large vessels issuing from them. For example, in so-called "blue babies," the pulmonary artery is narrowed and the ventricles are connected by an abnormal opening; in this cyanotic condition, the skin has a bluish tinge because the blood receives an insufficient amount of oxygen.

Formerly the expectation of life for such infants was extremely limited; with the advent of early diagnosis and improved techniques of hypothermia, surgery is often possible in the first week of life and the outlook for these infants is greatly improved.

Rheumatic heart disease was formerly one of the most serious forms of heart disease of childhood and adolescence, involving damage to the entire heart and its membranes. It usually followed attacks of rheumatic fever. Widespread use of antibiotics effective against the streptococcal bacterium that causes rheumatic fever has greatly reduced the incidence of this condition.

Myocarditis is inflammation or degeneration of the heart muscle. Although it is often caused by various diseases such as syphilis, goiter, endocarditis, or hypertension, myocarditis may appear as a primary disease in adults or as a degenerative disease of old age. It may be associated with dilation (enlargement due to weakness of the heart muscle) or with hypertrophy (overgrowth of the muscle tissue).

The major form of heart disease in Western countries is atherosclerosis. In this condition fatty deposits called plaque, composed of cholesterol and fats, build up on the inner wall of the coronary arteries. Gradual narrowing of the arteries throughout life restricts the blood flow to the heart muscles.

Symptoms of this restricted blood flow can include shortness of breath, especially during exercise, and a tightening pain in the chest called angina pectoris. The plaque may become large enough to completely obstruct the coronary artery, causing a sudden decrease in oxygen supply to the heart. Obstruction, also called occlusion, can occur when part of the plaque breaks away and lodges farther along in the artery, a process called thrombosis. These events are the major causes of heart attack, or myocardial infarction, which is often fatal. Persons who survive a heart attack must undergo extensive rehabilitation and risk a recurrence.

Development of fatty plaque is due partly to excessive intake of cholesterol and animal fats in the diet. A sedentary life-style is thought to promote atherosclerosis, and evidence suggests that physical exercise may help prevent heart disease. A striving, perfectionist temperament referred to as Type A personality has also been associated with increased risk of heart attacks, as has cigarette smoking. The occurrence of the heart attack itself is much more likely in persons who have high blood pressure. The actual event precipitating the attack may involve products secreted by platelets in the blood. This has led to clinical studies testing whether persons who have had a heart attack will be protected from a second infarction if they take drugs that block the action of platelets.

Many persons having severe angina because of atherosclerotic disease can be treated with drugs, such as propranolol and nitrates, which enable the heart to work more efficiently. Those who do not obtain relief with pharmacologic means can often be treated by a form of surgery called coronary bypass. In this procedure, which became established in the 1970s, a section of vein from the leg is sewn into the blocked coronary artery to form a bridge around the atherosclerotic region. In most recipients the operation relieves the pain of angina and in many persons it prevents a fatal heart attack. By 1986 more than 225,000 patients were undergoing these procedures each year in the U.S.

A second surgical procedure that was developed during the 1970s to treat atherosclerotic heart disease is balloon catheterization, technically called percutaneous transluminal coronary angioplasty. In this operation a wire with a balloon on the tip is inserted into an artery in the leg and threaded through the aorta into the coronary artery. When the balloon reaches the atherosclerotic area, it is inflated. The plaque is compressed and normal blood flow is reestablished. It is estimated that about one in six coronary bypass operations can be replaced by this less dangerous procedure.

During the 1970s and early 1980s it became apparent that a dramatic drop was occurring in mortality from atherosclerotic heart disease in developed countries. Although no definitive explanation for this decline has been given, public health officials have attributed it to widespread detection and treatment of high blood pressure and a decrease in the amount of animal fat in the average Western diet.

Some persons who die of apparent heart attacks exhibit no evidence of severe atherosclerosis. Research has shown that a decrease in blood flow to the heart can also be from vasospasm, the spontaneous contraction of an apparently healthy coronary artery. The existence of this phenomenon was documented in 1978 by Italian cardiologists. Vasospasm may contribute to some heart attacks brought on by atherosclerosis.

The immediate cause of death in many heart attacks, whether atherosclerosis is present or not, is ventricular fibrillation, also called cardiac arrest. This is a rapid ineffective beating of the ventricles. Normal heart rhythm can often be restored by a massive electric shock to the chest, a finding that has led to emergency rescue teams in many cities being trained in this technique.

Minor variations in the heart rhythm usually have little pathological significance. The heart rate responds to the demands of the body over such a wide range that variations are generally within normal limits. Severe defects, however, in the sinoatrial node or in the fibers that transmit impulses to the heart muscle can cause dizziness, faintness, and eventually death. The most serious of these conditions is called complete heart block. It can be corrected by insertion of an artificial pacemaker, a device that gives timed electric shocks to make the heart muscle contract in a regular pattern. More than 80,000 pacemakers are permanently implanted each year in the U.S. Most other arrhythmias are not dangerous except in persons with underlying heart disease. In these patients, especially those who have already had a heart attack, arrhythmias are treated with propranolol, lidocaine, and disopyramide.

Often found among older persons is cor pulmonale, or pulmonary heart disease, which usually is the result of a lung ailment, such as emphysema, or a disease affecting circulation to the lungs, such as arteriosclerosis of the pulmonary artery. Another condition found in older persons is congestive heart failure, in which the ventricles pump much less efficiently. The muscular walls of the ventricles enlarge with the effort to propel more of the blood into circulation, giving rise to the large, floppy hearts characteristic of this syndrome. Persons with this ailment have a reduced capacity for exercise. Their condition can often be improved with one of the derivatives of digitalis, which increases the pumping efficiency of the heart.

How DHEA can help the heart

As you can see, the ways in which a heart can become sick are extremely varied. So how can just one substance do so much to keep so many different problems away?

Let's look at some of these in greater detail.

First, it's important to understand that DHEA is not a "magic bullet." The latter is a term sometimes applied to drugs which go directly to a problem, act on that problem without affecting the rest of the body, and produce a minimum of side effects.

But the action of DHEA is not like that of a magic bullet. Rather, DHEA might more aptly be called a "magic blanket" because it interacts with a variety of physical mechanisms in the human body.

One of the substances in the human body affected by DHEA is insulin. Insulin is also a hormone and is secreted by the pancreas. Insulin regulates sugar levels in the blood stream, as well as starches. As you know, diabetics have lost the use of their pancreas's ability to produce insulin, thus wreaking havoc every time such an afflicted person eats certain amounts of sugars or starches.

Specifically, insulin is produced in a particular part of the pancreas called the islets of Langerhans. Like other proteins, insulin is partially digested if administered orally and hence must be injected into a muscle when used clinically. In the treatment of diabetes mellitus, which is caused by a deficiency of insulin production or by inhibition of its action on cells, insulin is often combined with protamine, which prolongs the period of absorption of the hormone. Insulin crystallized from the pancreas contains zinc, which also lengthens absorption. A preparation called protamine zinc insulin extends the hormone's action still further.

The older you are, the greater your chance of developing some kind of diabetes. More than 85 percent of all cases of diabetes afflict people over the age of 35. Interestingly, diabetes most often attacks people who are overweight, have a lot of unhealthy habits, and who have poor diets. And the older you get, the greater the chances that such bad habits are going to take a toll on the body.

Once again, we see that the condition of youth is like a get out of jail free card, providing the body with an almost magical resistance to not only disease, but bad behavior. A young college student, for example, can get drunk every weekend, smoke cigarettes, eat nothing but greasy burgers and french fries and even dabble in drugs — and still get up every morning, attend classes, work an outside job to help pay college expenses — and still feel good enough for even more hearty partying on the weekend.

All of this activity does not slow the powerful sex drive of the young college student, or their zest for strenuous and exiting activities, such as skiing, swimming, bike riding, playing sports, dancing and all the rest.

But as the college student ages, all of their bad habits begin to take a bigger and bigger toll on how the person feels. By age 30, the former college student is saying: "Jeez, I don't know how I did it! I used to work all day and party all night, now I have to be in bed by 10:30 and avoid alcohol, or I'm a zombie at work the next day. I'm sure not as young as I used to be!"

Part of the tremendous resistance to all that bad behavior may be the natural high levels of DHEA associated with the youthful body.

As the body ages, often insulin levels increase because, for some reason, the insulin which is being produced is less effective at regulating blood sugar and starch levels. For some reason, the body becomes resistant to insulin.

Insulin resistance very often leads to heart disease because it messes around with not only the blood, but the blood vessels. Insulin resistance can cause spasms of the blood vessels, cause them to become obstructed, and can inhibit the development of blood capillaries, which reduce the blood supply to all parts of the body, causing wide-spread damage.

Interestingly, the level of insulin in the body and the level of DHEA are directly related. As the level of DHEA goes down the harmful effects of the now unregulated insulin are allowed to move forward. Thus, it seems only common sense that replacing DHEA levels in the body as they decline with age will prevent not only diabetes, but the heart and blood vessel disease associated with insulin resistance.

Sticky Blood

The fact that blood can get sticky is a good thing. If blood did not have the ability to clot, any tiny cut could cause you to bleed to death. Blood clotting is nature's way of stopping the loss of too much blood due to cuts and other accidents.

On the other hand, clotting can get out of control. For some reason, some people have blood that wants to clot all the time, not just at those times when clotting is required. The result is "sluggish" blood, which can block arteries and slow the flow of blood to the heart and brain, causing heart disease and stroke, not to mention fatigue, poor brain function and other problems.

Tests with DHEA have shown that it can "unclog" overly sticky blood cells. When blood coagulants were added to a blood sample causing blood cells to clump together, adding DHEA reversed the action, thinning blood out and allowing it to move naturally. Thus, people who supplement their diets with DHEA may find that sticky blood problems will never afflict them, preventing a myriad of heart and other problems.

Cholesterol

We all know what a major problem cholesterol is. It clogs arteries, blocks heart valves, and contributes to the problems of obesity.

As you may know, medical researchers now make a distinction between "good cholesterol" and "bad cholesterol."

Cholesterol in fact is a complex alcohol constituent of all animal fats and oils. It can be activated to form vitamin D. Cholesterol is one of a group of compounds known as sterols and is related to such other sterols as the sex hormones and the hormones of the adrenal cortex.

A close relationship exists among levels of blood cholesterol in the body, those of other fats or lipids, and the development of atherosclerosis. In this disorder, plaques containing cholesterol are deposited on the walls of arteries, particularly those of small and medium size, reducing their inside diameter and the flow of blood. Clotting of blood, such as may occur in the coronary arteries to cause a heart attack, is most likely to develop at places where arterial walls are roughened by such plaques.

Although many foods, particularly dairy products and meat fat, contain cholesterol, the body also synthesizes this sterol from cholesterol-free substances. Nevertheless, investigation indicates that a cholesterol-rich diet causes abnormally high levels of cholesterol and the related fats and lipids in the blood. Evidence strongly indicates that persons with such high levels are more likely to develop atherosclerosis and heart attacks than those with lower levels.

As we said, doctors now recognize two distinct kinds of cholesterol-carrying proteins in the blood, called high-density (HDL) and low-density (LDL) lipoproteins. LDL is believed to promote atherosclerosis, and HDL may prevent this disease. Still, a 1984 study by the U.S. National Heart, Lung and Blood Institute found that high levels of LDL may also increase the risk of heart attacks and heart disease.

Finally, cholesterol and its derivatives are secreted through the oil glands of the skin to act as a lubricant and protective covering for the hair and skin. So cholesterol is not all bad, and furthermore, there are some kinds of cholesterol that are needed. After all your body makes this stuff for a reason. Without cholesterol, the human body would not be able to function!

Indeed, the most recent studies now show that having TOO LOW cholesterol may be as conducive to disease as high cholesterol. In a recent report on ABC News with Peter Jennings, scientists reported that people with cholesterol levels below 130 are generally less healthy than those with levels above 130, but below 200. Thus, there may be an "optimum" cholesterol level to maintain, but exactly what that level is has yet to be determined.

The point is, taking DHEA may regulate the proper level in each person automatically. DHEA seems able to lower cholesterol levels because it enhances the ability of the liver to use lipids properly. Rather than struggling to regulate both HDL and LDL through manipulation of diet, a simple tablet of DHEA taken every day will get the job done for you automatically — although more study is still needed to prove this conclusively.

DHEA and the Battle of the Bulge

Medical researchers and millions of Americans have long been searching for the ultimate diet pill. That's because obesity has become a major health problem in our society today. Obesity is characterized by storage of excessive amounts of fat in adipose tissue beneath the skin and within other organs, including muscles. All mammals store body fat; in normal women 25 percent, and in normal men 15 percent, of body weight is stored as fat.

Deposition of fat, which has twice the potential energy of carbohydrate or protein, is a way of storing energy for times of future need. Storage of greatly increased amounts of fat, however, is associated with impairment of health. Data from insurance company records show that persons who are 30 percent or more overweight run measurably increased risks of disease, notably diabetes, cardiovascular and gallbladder disease, and arthritis, and often encounter complications in surgery.

Obesity is only rarely caused by disturbances of the endocrine system. It is not inherited, nor do fat babies necessarily grow up to be fat adults. Obesity is a result of taking in more energy in food than one uses in activity. Scientists have found that both obese and normal-weight people go on eating binges, but people of normal weight reduce their intake afterward to compensate, whereas obese people do not. Besides excess eating, obesity can also be caused by reduced activity, and this often occurs in persons who are sedentary or bedridden.

Many approaches to weight loss have been tried in obese people, with only limited success. Diet pills, containing the stimulant drug dextroamphetamine or one of its derivatives, became popular in the 1950s, but the Food and Drug Administration issued a series of warnings to physicians that they did not work and could be habit-forming, and their use declined. Many complex diets have been promoted for weight loss, but no scientific evidence exists that they are effective for grossly obese people. One form of diet developed to provide nourishment for hospitalized people, the liquid protein diet, was marketed commercially until 1979, when it was found that several people had died while using this mixture as a sole source of nutrition. The mixture upset the natural balance of sodium and potassium in the body, leading to impaired heart function.

Recently the extremely popular diet pill combination known as Phen-Fen has been discovered to cause severe cardio-pulmonary dysfunction, and even death do to heart damage.

What this all gets down to is that medical science simply has not been able to find a safe, simple and effective medication which can help people bring their body's metabolism under control, making the body stop storing fat in excessive amounts, and maintain a proper balance of fat-to muscle ratio.

Exciting new research suggests that DHEA may be the "Holy Grail" of fat fighting supplements we all have been looking for. As far back as the late 1970s, medical researchers were giving DHEA to obese mice, and were surprised to discovery that the hormone seemed to literally "melt" that fat right out of the rodent's bodies. Furthermore, the weight loss occurred even if the mice were allowed to maintain their high fat diets and the other bad habits they were induced to have, such as lack of exercise. DHEA seemed able to produce optimum weight levels in mice no matter what their eating or exercise habits.

After these positive and promising results with mice, many veterinarians decided to try DHEA on dogs. As it turns out, man's best friend has as many problems with obesity as do their masters, mostly for all the same reasons — a plentiful supply of hard-to-resist fatty foods and little daily exercise.

Again, the results were spectacular. Several thousand overweight dogs were placed on a daily regimen of DHEA, all relatively high doses, and some 68 percent of the animals lost weight, and returned to a healthy, optimum weight level.

The dogs that did not respond well to DHEA therapy were those that were considered morbidly obese, those that were so heavy as to be beyond the point of no return, no matter what kind of steps were taken to reduce their weight.

The evidence obtained from mice and dogs seems to strongly indicate, however, that DHEA may be one of the best weight loss pills available to medical science. Can it work the same in human beings?

All indications are that it can. Here's why: DHEA seems to strongly effect the way the body breaks down, burns and uses food. It seems that DHEA makes the body less efficient at energy conservation — that's right LESS EFFECTIVE.

That's important because when the body is good at conserving energy, that means it is good at storing up fat.

Mother Nature designed the human body with a strategy to get it through those lean times when food was not plentiful. Before the invention of agriculture and modern food storage methods, human beings ate well in those times — most likely summer months — when food was plentiful, and had to scrounge and conserve during the seasons of scarcity. If the body was not good at storing up fat for a rainy day, so to speak, it would have little chance of getting through the months of food scarcity.

These days famine is all but unheard of in the developed world. Food is plentiful year-round, and not just food, but lots of fatty foods. So while the body is programmed to conserve energy and save all the fat it can, just in case a famine breaks out, the result in modern society is lots of fat intake and lots of fat storage as a continuous process — the frequent result is a lot of very fat people!

DHEA makes the human body less active at storing energy and saving fat cells. DHEA also seems to block the formation of fatty acids. Furthermore, DHEA seems to make animals (including humans) WANT to eat less - that is, crave less food. That's because your brain is reading your body's energy level as "normal." After all it is your brain which makes you hungry. Your brain monitors the body's level of nutrition, blood sugar level, etc. If the brain receives a low blood sugar message, it prompts you to eat something to bring the blood sugar level back up to normal.

Many people crave high fat and sweet foods. That's because the body's metabolism is telling the brain that it needs more fat and quick energy, even when it can easily get by without it. DHEA would appear to change that. Lab animals who are "addicted" to fatty foods change their preferences to leaner, low-fat food when they are given daily doses of DHEA. The brain is demanding a different diet because the "read-out" from the body's hormone messenger system has adjusted its food requirements.

Much more study needs to be done, but DHEA, because of its relative safety, and because it regulates a broad range of body chemistry activities, does more than just address obesity problems in human beings. It takes care of a broad range of body chemistry parameters, all of which can lead to people getting fat.

The only drawback to DHEA as a diet pill is that very high doses were needed to produce desired results in dogs and lab animals. Still, with further research, and perhaps by using DHEA in combination with other drugs, such as Prozac or Zoloft, DHEA may be the ultimate diet pill of the future.

DHEA and Menopause

Menopause is a major hormonal event in the lives of women. For many women, this means emotional upheaval. Most often, it's not a positive change, at least it's difficult for most women to feel positive as the hormones of their body began to play tournament hockey in their blood streams.

Menopause is the period in a woman's life when menstruation ceases, and she is no longer able to bear children. Natural menopause results from changes in the ovaries and in glands that produce the hormones (primarily estrogen) that control the menstrual cycle. In most women, this decline in estrogen production occurs between the ages of 45 and 50. (Recent research indicates that men, as they age, do not experience hormonal declines comparable to those in menopausal women.) Surgical removal or other destruction of the ovaries can produce premature menopause at any age.

Many women undergo menopause without difficulty. But many experience hot flashes and sweats; changes in the vaginal lining that produce dryness, burning, itching, and pain during sexual intercourse; and osteoporosis, a thinning of the bone associated with an increased risk of fracture. These problems, caused by hormonal deficiencies or imbalances, are effectively controlled or prevented by estrogen-replacement therapy. Because postmenopausal estrogen use has been linked to an increased risk of cancer of the lining of the uterus, however, its use in treating symptoms of menopause has become controversial. Given the current state of knowledge, no general recommendation can be made; the decision about its use should be made by the woman and her doctor.

At one time, depression and other emotional problems were considered more common in a woman's life during menopause; this notion is now being questioned. Menopause nevertheless is a psychological as well as a physical milestone in the aging process, and such milestones sometimes produce varying degrees of stress.

What about DHEA and menopause? It seems that estrogen is the primary hormone at play here, and for certain we'll have more to say about estrogen in the section of this book which takes an in-depth look at estrogen.

As it turns out, there is already a body of research on DHEA and women experiencing menopause. Marketed under the name praterone in Europe, doctors over there have been treating women for menopause-related depression with DHEA. Also, other menopausal symptoms are being treated with combinations of DHEA, estrogen and other hormones.

You see, DHEA is a substance out of which estrogen is made. DHEA is a vital building block of estrogen.

Today, there is a lot of anecdotal evidence that taking only DHEA, and skipping estrogen replacement therapy, may be all the treatment women need to deal with the problems associated with menopause. In fact, in several completed clinical studies, DHEA seems to offer all the same benefits of estrogen replacement therapy, without the risks of the same.

In addition to relieving or entirely eliminating the most common symptoms of menopause, the DHEA treatment of the women in the test group also seemed to reduce blood insulin levels and blood sugar levels. This is further evidence that DHEA may be an extremely effective deterrent to diabetes in older people. Along with a reduction in risk for diabetes goes reduction in risk for heart disease. That's because high insulin rates, as we have discussed, play a major role in damaging heart valves, arteries and other conduits of the blood.

Many menopausal women experience weight gain, but again, in the studies completed, women who took DHEA saw their weight reduced or normalized, even while menopause continued. At the same time, the muscle tone of the women improved, and the fat-to-muscle ratio was balanced to optimum levels. In addition to optimum weight, the rapid bone thinning that is associated with menopause did not occur with women who took DHEA at the onset of their menopause, and, in fact, most of the women saw an increase in their bone density. This in and of itself is a major boone to women who struggle to maintain their calcium levels and stave off the crippling effects of osteoporosis.

Furthermore, DHEA in menopausal women caused a balancing effect in cholesterol levels, which helps explain the weight loss and lowering of heart disease factors. Finally, DHEA seemed to greatly improve another common symptom of menopause — vaginal drying, also known as vaginal atrophy. It's caused by a reduction in the secretion of lubricants which protect the vaginal walls, both during sex and nonsex periods. Overall, this has the effect of improving enjoyment and safety of sexual activity in the post-menopausal life of women.

What DHEA did not do in the above studies is also important. It did not stimulate the growth of unwanted vaginal tissues, as does estrogen therapy in some cases. It also did not stimulate the growth of the uterine lining.

The three to five days the egg takes to reach the uterus after being released by the ovary is known as the woman's fertile period. If fertilization does occur, the fertilized egg attaches itself to the enriched uterine lining and pregnancy continues. Menstruation does not occur during pregnancy, and a missed period is often the first indication of pregnancy a woman notices. If fertilization does not occur, the lining of the uterus does not receive the hormones it needs to continue the thickening process. Thus, the uterine lining breaks down and is discharged from the body during menstruation.

Before menopause, the building up of the lining of the vaginal walls and the lining of the uterus is a necessary function. This process prepares the uterus to receive a fertilized egg, if one should be made available. Menstruation is triggered by the hormone progesterone.

Progesterone is a hormone formed by the granulosa cells of the corpus luteum of the ovary. The corpus luteum is a structure in the ovary that develops at the site where a mature egg was released at ovulation. Therefore the level of progesterone rises in the second half of the menstrual cycle. If the released ovum is not fertilized, production of progesterone falls just before the onset of the next menstrual cycle and the corpus luteum degenerates. Progesterone was isolated and crystallized by three independent groups of investigators in 1934. It is a steroid hormone, a compound possessing the same chemical nucleus as the female estrogenic hormones and the male androgenic hormones, as well as cholesterol and adrenal steroid hormones. The principal function of progesterone is the preparation of the mucous membrane of the uterus for the reception of the ovum. The hormone also stimulates the formation of saclike structures in the lacteal glands in preparation for their function of producing milk, and inhibits the release in the pituitary of prolactin hormone.

But after menopause, the progesterone trigger ceases, while the build-up of the uterine lining can continue. The result is often cancer. Doctors often attempt to counter this outcome by prescribing progesterone for women, which makes them continue experiencing menstruation, even though they no longer have any eggs to slough off. This kind of hormone therapy has its drawbacks as well, however. Progesterone therapy produces PMS symptoms in many women, including bloating, depression, irritability and mood swings. Because of this, researchers are looking for alternatives to progesterone therapy as a way to counterbalance estrogen replacement therapy.

Once again, researchers may have found their answer in DHEA because it appears to eliminate the need for estrogen therapy altogether, while at the same time providing all the benefits thereof.

DHEA and Wrinkles

Probably more than anything else, wrinkled, leathery skin is associated with old age. This is a bit ironic, since wrinkled skin is not life threatening in and of itself. Compared to thinning bones, a bad heart or anemic blood, for example, a few wrinkles are slight problems. But the fact that wrinkled skin makes a person LOOK so old makes it a major consideration in this whole question of maintaining youth.

Restoring the smoothness and eliminating the wrinkles of the face can make a person look 20-30 years younger instantly, even though nothing else about the person had changed. While in this case beauty can truly be said to be skin deep, improving the look and feel of the skin should not be taken lightly. In order for a person to feel young, the appearance of youth carries enormous psychological weight.

Also, the skin is important because it forms a protective barrier against the action of physical, chemical, and bacterial agents on the deeper tissues and contains the special end organs for the various sensations commonly grouped as the sense of touch. Through the activity of its sweat glands and blood vessels, it is important in maintaining body temperature. One square inch of skin contains up to 15 ft of blood vessels, which have as one of their functions the regulation of body temperature.

When the body temperature rises, heat is lost because of vascular dilation and increased blood flow to the skin surface. When the temperature is low, blood vessels constrict to reduce blood flow and subsequent heat loss through the skin. Each square inch of skin also contains hundreds of sweat glands that are controlled by a heat regulation center in the brain. These glands secrete moisture, which evaporates, cools the body surface, and helps maintain normal body temperature. In this capacity the skin acts as an excretory organ. The skin is elastic, and except for a few areas such as the palms, soles, and ears, is loosely attached to the underlying tissues.

The color of the skin varies normally with the amount of pigment deposited in the skin cells as governed by heredity and by exposure to sunlight. The color also varies in disease because of difference in pigment, as in Addison's disease, or because of pigmented substances carried to it by the blood as in jaundice. In certain places the outer layers of the skin are modified to produce the hair and nails. The skin varies in thickness from 0.02 of an inch on the eyelids to 0.17 of an inch or more on the palms and soles.

In structure the skin is composed of two distinct layers. The outer layer, called the epidermis or cuticle, is several cells thick and has an external, horny layer of dead cells that is constantly shed from the surface and replaced from below by a basal layer of cells, the stratum germinativum. The inner layer, called the corium or dermis, is composed of a network of collagen and elastic fibers, blood vessels, nerves, fat lobules, and the bases of hair follicles and sweat glands. The interface between the epidermis and dermis is extremely irregular and consists of a succession of papillae, or fingerlike projections, which are smallest where the skin is thin and longest in the skin of the palms and soles. The papillae of the palms and soles are associated with elevations of the epidermis which produce ridges that are the basis for fingerprint identification. Each papilla contains either a capillary loop of blood vessels or a specialized nerve ending. The vascular loops, supplying nutrients to the epidermis, outnumber the neural papillae by about four to one.

Sweat, or sudoriferous, glands are found on every part of the body. They are numerous on the palms and soles but relatively sparse on the skin of the back. Each gland consists of coiled tubules that are situated in the subcutaneous tissue and a duct that extends through the dermis and forms a convoluted spiral through the epidermis. Sebaceous glands, saclike glands that secrete the sebum that lubricates and softens the skin, open into the hair follicles a short distance below the surface of the epidermis.

The skin is prone to diseases from external as well as internal causes. Inflammation of the skin, or dermatitis, may often result from exposure to physically or chemically irritating substances in industry, from contact with such vegetable poisons as the toxin of poison ivy, or from sunburn, overexposure to the ultraviolet rays of the sun. Infection of the skin with pyogenic streptococci gives rise to impetigo and erysipelas, and infections of the skin spread throughout the body, as in syphilis, smallpox, and tuberculosis; general systemic disorders may produce skin symptoms, as in measles, scarlet fever, and chicken pox. Foreign proteins, or proteins to which the body is unduly sensitive, may affect the skin by producing hives, or wheals, whether the protein reaches the skin through the bloodstream or whether it is applied directly to the skin. Patients are often tested by placing a small amount of the protein on a small scratch in the skin; sensitivity is indicated by the appearance of a wheal. Eczema, formerly considered the most common skin disease, is now regarded as a symptom of any of a variety of conditions, including external local irritations, disorders of the blood, and allergy. Other skin affections include tumors, sebaceous cysts (wens), ulcers and pigmentations that are congenital or are caused by disorders of the internal secretions, and melanoma.

What can DHEA do about all this, including the strictly cosmetic appearance of the skin? Dermatologists now believe that the function of the sebaceous glands is directly related to DHEA. High DHEA means high sebum amounts in the skin. Too much sebum causes acne, which is why teen-agers with surging hormones levels tend to suffer from a lot of problems with acne. As they grow older, DHEA falls off and the skin dries out and acne clears up. While it's nice to get rid of acne, the skin goes to far in the other direction, losing sebum and getting dry and wrinkled.

The key is not to simply apply a moisturizer to the surface of the skin, as do most cosmetics on the market. Rather, the sebaceous glands themselves must be restored to their youthful activity. Skin creams containing DHEA have been shown to do just that. Those who have applied DHEA to their skin via a topical application find that wrinkles disappear and that skin feels better and softer.

Interestingly, the subject of dry skin has a connection with another common problem of aging —

dry eyes. Like the skin, the eyes are also lubricated by moisture producing glands called the meibomiam glands. These are a close cousin to the sabaceous glands of the skin. Thus, medical researchers reasoned that if DHEA skin creams could jump start the sebaceous glands in the skin, perhaps it could also work its magic on the meibomiam glands.

The first experiments were done with dogs. Eye drops containing DHEA were applied to several thousand aging dogs with dry eyes, and the results were positive. The eyes of the dogs seemed to return to their youthful clarity and normal moisture levels. Limited studies have already been completed on humans with similar results. Even elderly people who were no longer able to wear contact lenses because of dry eyes found they could toss away their regular eye glasses and go back to contacts after using DHEA enhanced eye drops.

Again, such medication goes beyond the mere surface treatment of applying over-the-counter eye drops, which contain only a saline solution that puts moisture at the surface of the eye. Real tear drops are not water, but actually a complex mixture of water mixed with natural body fats, which can only be manufactured from within by the meibomiam glands. DHEA drops stimulate these glands into working at their nominal, youthful level.

DHEA and Autoimmune Diseases

Scientists are looking to DHEA as a possible weapon against one of the most difficult classes of human illnesses called autoimmune diseases.

These are illnesses in which the body, for some reason, literally begins to attack itself. The immune system reacts to normal components of the body as if they were foreign substances and produces antibodies against them.

Antibodies are manufactured by cells called lymphocytes. It is thought that, during development of the embryo, lymphocytes capable of reacting with the body's own tissues are somehow inactivated so that the self is distinguished from the nonself and is not destroyed by antibodies. Self-reactive lymphocytes can still be found in some adults, however, which suggests that they are actively suppressed in some way rather than eliminated.

Another mechanism for protecting components of the self from destruction is sequestration during early development. Mature sperm cells, for example, do not appear until after the immune system has matured and are then automatically separated from the bloodstream. After vasectomy, these cells enter the bloodstream, where they can provoke formation of antibodies against themselves.

One theory to explain autoimmune disease proposes that suppression of reaction against the self is disrupted when viruses infect the antibody-forming cells. In the infectious form of mononucleosis, in which lymphocytes are invaded by a virus, antibodies against a variety of body tissues are found in the bloodstream. Rheumatic heart disease is believed to be a result of childhood infection by streptococcal bacteria, which have a surface molecular arrangement identical to one found in heart muscle; antibodies formed against the bacteria can also damage the heart.

In most other autoimmune diseases the cause of antibody formation is unknown. Persons with myasthenia gravis make an antibody that blocks the transmission of nerve impulses to muscle; this causes the muscle weakness and breathing difficulty associated with the disease. In autoimmune hemolytic anemia, the red blood cells are destroyed by autoantibodies. Persons with lupus erythematosus make antibodies that attack cell components, including genetic material. Clumps of matter formed by antibodies bound to the cell components can damage the kidneys. The blood of some persons with arthritis contains rheumatoid factor, an antibody that binds to other antibodies in the blood; whether this factor also causes the joint injury of arthritis is not known.

Lupus, arthritis, and the skin diseases scleroderma and dermatomyositis are called collagen diseases because of the damage the associated antibodies cause to connective tissue, which is made up of collagen.

A few severe cases of diabetes are caused by an antibody that destroys insulin-forming cells in the pancreas. Another antibody attacks the thyroid gland, producing chronic thyroiditis. Addison's disease in some cases may result from autoimmune destruction of the adrenal gland.

One of the most intensively studied autoimmune diseases is multiple sclerosis. In this illness the myelin sheath covering the spinal cord is destroyed, leading to difficulty in walking and other movements. The damage in multiple sclerosis is not produced by an autoantibody but by a lymphocyte that reacts directly with the protective sheath.

Autoantibodies are often found in the blood of older persons who have no disease, a phenomenon that is not understood.

Treatment of autoimmune diseases usually entails therapy with steroids, which suppress the immune system. Currently under investigation is a procedure called plasmapheresis, in which the patient's blood is passed through a machine that removes gamma globulin, the blood fraction that contains antibodies.

One of the most common autoimmune diseases is Lupus Erythematosus, or just lupus for short. This disease is often identified by the characteristic "butterfly rash" it causes on the face, although it's main effect on the body involves the internal organs.

Lupus strikes women nine times as often as men. The disease is thought to be a result of the malfunctioning of the immune system. The blood of a lupus patient contains antibodies against many normal tissue components. Damage caused by these antibodies produces arthritic joint disease, heart damage, shortness of breath, and impaired kidney function. Lupus follows an irregular course of remissions and flare-ups, but is often incapacitating. Treatment is rest and drugs — nonsteroidal anti-inflammatories, such as aspirin, or corticosteroids, but these do not usually halt the disease's progression.

Can DHEA help where these more traditional drugs have failed? Several small studies indicate that DHEA may indeed hold part of the clue to conquering this agonizing condition.

In one recent study, a group of women with mild to moderate cases of lupus were given daily doses of DHEA, while another control group were given a placebo. After several months, more than 65 percent of the women who received DHEA showed clear improvement in their condition. The women who received only blanks showed no improvement. While one-third of the women did not improve at all, the fact that most of them did is an important and significant finding. Additionally, a smaller percentage of the women felt they were "completely cured" of their lupus by DHEA.

Just how DHEA works to counter lupus in still not known, but medical researchers theorize that it has a lot to do with the extremely complex immune system of the human body. The body's immune system is regulated by a myriad of hormonal interactions. Such a complex process lends itself well to the power of DHEA since its action is that of regulating the process of most of the prominent hormones, bringing them all into balance and acting in accord with each other. There is still much research to be done on DHEA and autoimmune diseases, but the future looks promising.

DHEA and Burns

Almost 2 million people suffer serious burns in the United States each year. Some 115,000 are hospitalized and 12,000 die of this hellish kind of injury every year.

How bad a burn is depends on how deep it goes, the area it covers, and the age of the victim. Burns are classified by depth as first, second, and third degree. First-degree burns cause redness and pain. Second-degree burns are marked by blisters. In third-degree burns, both the epidermis and dermis are destroyed, and underlying tissue may also be damaged. The extent of a burn is expressed as the percent of total skin surface which is injured. Persons under 1 year and over 40 years old have a higher mortality rate than those between 2 and 39 for burns of similar depth and extent. Inhalation of smoke from a fire significantly increases mortality.

Thermal destruction of the skin permits infection, which is the most common cause of death for extensively burned persons. Body fluids and minerals are lost through the wound. The lungs, heart, liver, and kidneys are affected by the infection and fluid loss.

First aid for most burns is cool water applied soon after the burn. Application of home remedies should be avoided. Burns of 15 percent of the body surface or less are usually treated in hospital emergency rooms by removing dead tissue, dressing with antibiotic cream, and administering oral pain medication. Burns of 15 to 25 percent often require hospitalization to provide intravenous fluids and avoid complications. Burns of more than 25 percent are usually treated in specialized burn centers where aggressive surgical management is directed toward early skin grafting and avoidance of such complications as dehydration, pneumonia, kidney failure, and infection. Pain control with intravenous narcotics is frequently required. The markedly increased metabolic rate of severely burned patients requires high-protein nutritional supplements given by mouth and intravenously. Extensive scarring of deep burns may cause disfigurement and limitation of joint motion. Plastic surgery is often required to reduce the effects of the scars.

Now DHEA may be another important weapon in medical science's effort to treat burn victims. Doctors have long observed that burns have a powerful negative effect on the body's ability to heal itself. Thus, burns in effect are a kind of autoimmune problem because they dampen the healing mechanism of the body. That's where DHEA can help. The hormone can give burn victims an immune boost, stimulating the body to work harder at healing burns.

Tests on animals which have been burned already indicate that DHEA speeds the healing of burns. Doctors will undoubtedly be taking a much closer look at DHEA as a new weapon against one of the most common and painful kinds of injury in the world.

DHEA Conclusions

In this section we have examined a broad range of applications for DHEA and its many exciting possibilities to prevent disease, to heal existing disease, and to restore aged bodies back to youthful levels of existence.

DHEA truly does seem to be a key in keeping the body young. It shows potential to become a class of treatment that rivals the invention of antibiotics and immunizations, which added decades to the average life expectancy of all human beings.

Just as antibiotic and vaccines almost instantly increased the average life expectancy of age 49 in the year 1900 to the average of age 75 we all enjoy today, DHEA and other super hormones may give us another 30, 40 or 50 additional years of normal life on this planet earth.

Speaking of other hormones, let's move on now to the other super hormones, and examine how they can help people live longer lives, and lives of higher quality.

NOTES

_____

_____

_____

_____

_____

_____

_____

Chapter 2

Pregnenolone: The Mind Hormone

E veryone knows that old people have trouble with their memories. We all accept it as "natural" that the older you get, the poorer your mental capacity becomes. Many even consider it a kind of affectionate aspect of old age. We all picture in our minds the sweet, elderly grandfather or grandmother with their white hair and mental slips that give them a child-like adorability.

But losing your mind is never a good thing. It also is not natural. Senility is a disease in the truest sense of the word. It is a condition that robs you of your quality of life. It impairs your ability to work at jobs that require mental acuity and alertness.

Senile dementia, as it is more properly called, affects about 10 percent of all people over the age of 65. Although about 20 percent of these cases may be due to treatable causes such as toxic drug reactions, most cases are what is known as Alzheimer's disease.

Senile dementia begins with failing attention and memory, loss of mathematical ability, irritability and loss of sense of humor, and poor orientation in space and time. Alzheimer's disease is relentlessly progressive and leads to death in 5 to 15 years. Examinations of the brains of persons who have died of Alzheimer's disease show characteristic twisted fibers, called neurofibrillary tangles, in certain areas of the brain, and cores of abnormal protein, called neuritic plaques, interspersed among nerve cells.

One of the keys to stopping all these bad things from happening to an aging brain is the hormone pregnenolone. Many scientists consider this hormone the true key to maintaining a healthy mind late into life.

Pregnenolone seems to not only aid the proper functioning of the memory, but also the critical thinking aspect of the mind, and even our mental feelings of happiness and well-being.

Just what is pregnenolone? This hormone comes from the substance we all know as cholesterol. As we have said earlier in this book, most people consider cholesterol to be a bad thing. That's not hard to understand considering all the constant media noise about the dangers of high cholesterol levels and the many health problems it causes for the human body.

But it's important to acknowledge the fact that cholesterol is not all bad. There is "good" cholesterol and "bad" cholesterol, but medical researchers now think that there really is no such thing as bad cholesterol, only too much of a good thing. Truly, life itself would be impossible without cholesterol. Additionally, researchers have now concluded that too little cholesterol in the blood can lead to a whole host of other kinds of diseases, including mental illness. A recent and significant study showed that a large percentage of prisoners had low cholesterol levels. Apparently, too little cholesterol in the blood is a major factor in anti-social behavior, including violent anger and moderate to severe depression.

Cholesterol is needed by the body to produce vitamin D, which is a vital part of many bodily functions, including the body's ability to absorb calcium. Vitamin D also aids in the manufacturing of myelin, the sheath of material that coats the nerves. Those people who suffer from degenerative diseases such as multiple sclerosis are unable to produce myelin, and also have their existing myelin erode from its position on the nerves. The result is a loss of muscle control, life-time of crippling weakness and loss of use of the most fundamental bodily movements.

So cholesterol is broken down into the hormone pregnenolone and other hormones, including DHEA. Pregnenolone is sometimes called the "mother hormone" because other hormones such as DHEA and estrogen and testosterone come from it.

Pregnenolone is manufactured in the brain and by the adrenal cortex, glands positioned on top of the kidneys. The two parts of the gland, the inner portion, or medulla, and the outer portion, or cortex, are like separate endocrine organs. They are composed of different types of tissue and perform different functions. The adrenal medulla, composed of chromaffin, secretes the hormone epinephrine, also called adrenaline, in response to stimulation of the sympathetic nervous system at times of stress. The medulla also secretes the hormone norepinephrine, which plays a role in maintaining normal blood circulation. The hormones of the medulla are called catecholamines. Unlike the cortex, the medulla can be removed without endangering the life of an individual.

The adrenal outer layer, or cortex, secretes about 30 steroid hormones, but only a few are secreted in significant amounts. Aldosterone, one of the most important hormones, regulates the salt and water balance in the body. Cortisone and hydrocortisone are also vital; they regulate fat, carbohydrate, and protein metabolism.

Also secreted are adrenal sex steroids, which have a minor influence on the reproductive system. Modified glucocorticoids, now produced synthetically, are superior to naturally secreted steroids for treatment of Addison's disease and other disorders.

Like DHEA, pregnenolone production drops off in the human body as it ages. By the time most people hit age 75, their bodies are producing about 60 percent less of the hormone than they were at age 30. This is significant because, as we said, pregnenolone is the "parent" to other vital hormones in the body. Lose your pregnenolone and you lose a lot of other vital, youth enhancing hormones.

Pregnenolone can be purchased at any health food store without a prescription from a doctor.

Pregnenolone and Memory

Before we look at how pregnenolone aids the memory, let's take a closer look at what memory is.

Memory is basically the process of storing and retrieving information in the brain. Naturally, this process is important for learning and thinking. <u>Four different types of remembering are ordinarily distinguished by psychologists: recollection, recall, recognition, and relearning</u>. Recollection involves the reconstruction of events or facts on the basis of partial cues, which serve as reminders. Recall is the active and unaided remembering of something from the past. Recognition refers to the ability to correctly identify previously encountered stimuli as familiar. Relearning may show evidence of the effects of memory; material that is familiar is often easier to learn a second time than it would be if it were unfamiliar.

The course of forgetting over time has been studied extensively by psychologists. Most often a rapid forgetting occurs at first, followed by a decreasing rate of loss. Improvement in the amount of material retained, however, can be achieved by practicing active recall during learning, by periodic reviews of the material, and by overlearning the material beyond the point of bare mastery. A mechanical technique devised to improve memory is mnemonics, involving the use of associations and various devices to remember particular facts. Four traditional explanations of forgetting have been provided. One is that memory traces fade naturally over time as a result of organic processes occurring in the nervous system, although little evidence for this notion exists. A second is that memories become systematically distorted or modified over time. A third is that new learning often interferes with or replaces old learning, a phenomenon known as retroactive inhibition. Finally, some forgetting may be motivated by the needs and wishes of the individual, as in repression.

Little is known about the physiology of memory storage in the brain. Some researchers suggest that memories are stored at specific sites, and others that memories involve widespread brain regions working together; both processes may in fact be involved.

Theorists also propose that different storage mechanisms exist for short-term and long-term memories, and that if memories are not transferred from the former to the latter they will be lost. Animal studies indicate that structures in the brain's limbic system have different memory functions. For example, one circuit through the hippocampus and thalamus may be involved in spatial memories, whereas another, through the amygdala and thalamus, may be involved in emotional memories. Research also suggests that ìskillî memories are stored differently from intellectual memories.

In general, memories are less clear and detailed than perceptions, but occasionally a remembered image is complete in every detail. This phenomenon, known as eidetic imagery, is usually found in children, who sometimes project the image so completely that they can spell out an entire page of writing in an unfamiliar language that they have seen for a short time.

To date, many drugs have been developed to aid memory in those people who are having trouble with it. Unfortunately, few of these drugs are effective and they generally have a lot of negative side effects.

But new research indicates that the very best memory drugs may be the natural hormone pregnenolone. Extensive studies have already been performed on mice in a laboratory setting. Mice who were taught specific tasks, such as finding their way through mazes, choosing specific doors, etc. learned to perform these tasks with spectacular efficiency when give injections of pregnenolone. They also could remember their tasks weeks later with far better clarity than those who did not receive pregnenolone injections.

Can it work the same miracles on human memory. As it turns out, pregnenolone's effect on the improvement of memory has been understood by medical researchers for more than 50 years! The University of Massachusetts tested subjects on specific memory tasks and found that pregnenolone vastly improved the performance of human memory in a variety of laboratory testing situations. Pregnenolone was also given to people in the "real world" including pilots and factory workers, and again, those who took the hormone showed definite improvement in how they were able to perform their jobs. Not only were they able to perform their work better, they also reported feeling less stress, and a generally greater sense of joy and satisfaction with how they felt about their work and lives.

It is unknown why after such positive results science did not look further into pregnenolone as a memory enhancer. Most likely, there was a lot of general concern about side effects and a lot of unknowns since knowledge of the body's chemistry was far less advanced than it is today. One negative side-effect, for example, was an increased feeling of stress and anxiety on behalf of some of the subjects. This makes sense because pregnenolone boosts the body's production of corticosteroids, the primary stress causing hormones.

Today, scientists are taking a closer look at pregnenolone and its effect on not only memory, but a variety of human thought processes.

At the St. Louis University School of Medicine, doctors administered pregnenolone and a placebo to two groups of older men and women. Three hours after taking the hormone, they were asked to perform a battery of standard memory tests, and other tests involving use of the critical thinking factors of the brain. Those given pregnenolone showed improvement, but not improvement across the board. Amazingly, the differences varied by sex. Men tended to work visual spatial tasks better and women improved in their verbal recall skills. As we will later see, the reason for the difference between male and female reaction to pregnenolone probably has a lot to do with the fact that testosterone, the male hormone, and estrogen, the female hormone, are derived from pregnenolone. Thus. men who receive pregnenolone supplements probably favor using it as eventual testosterone while women favor it as an estrogen derivative.

Pregnenolone, Prozac and the biochemistry of Depression

Perhaps America's No. 1 disease, depression afflicts as many as 20 of every 100 people. Many of these people suffer from a number of different but significant depressive symptoms at any one time. Also, more than 30 percent of all people can expect to suffer from at least some kind of depression over the course of a lifetime. The disorder strikes men and women of all ages, in all segments of society, but most studies indicate that women are more prone to depression than men.

Depression is characterized by feelings of worthlessness, guilt, sadness, helplessness, and hopelessness. In contrast to normal sadness or the grief accompanying the loss of a loved one, clinical depression is persistent and severe. It is accompanied by a variety of related symptoms, including disturbances in sleep and eating, loss of initiative, self-punishment, withdrawal and inactivity, and loss of pleasure.

Psychologists divide depression into two major categories. In both, the predominant symptom is a disturbance in mood. One form of the disorder, depressive disorder, is marked only by episodes of depression. The other, bipolar or manic depressive illness, is characterized by alternating depressed and manic episodes.

In major depression or the depressed phase of bipolar illness, a depressed mood predominates, although the patient may not be aware of feeling sad. Typically, he or she loses all interest in and withdraws from usual activities. Symptoms include sleep disturbances, loss of appetite or greatly increased appetite, inability to concentrate or to make decisions, slowed thinking and decreased energy, feelings of worthlessness, guilt, hopelessness, and helplessness, diminished sexual interest; and recurrent thoughts of suicide and death, sometimes leading to actual suicide.

In the manic phase of bipolar illness, the patient's mood can be elevated, expansive, or irritable. Behavior is bizarre and sometimes obnoxious. Other symptoms include excessive talkativeness, racing thoughts, and grandiose ideas; greatly increased social, sexual, and work activity; distractibility; loss of judgment; and a decreased need for sleep.

Both depressive and bipolar disorders run in families. Almost certainly a predisposition to these disorders is genetically transmitted. Thus, the risk of a depressive disorder is greater in the families of depressive patients than in the population at large. The higher proportion of depression in women may be biologically induced, or it may be that women learn social roles that favor feelings of helplessness. Because women in trouble are more likely to seek help than men, statistics reporting a higher incidence of depression among women than among men may be explained, at least in part, by an underdiagnosis of depression in men.

Studies have suggested that genetic predisposition to depression may be linked with an abnormal sensitivity to the neurotransmitter acetylcholine. Receptors for acetylcholine have been found to occur in excessive numbers in the skin of a number of patients suffering from depressive disorders.

Fortunately, depressive disorders are considered among the most treatable in psychiatry. The usual treatment in modern practice involves administration of a drug plus supportive psychotherapy. Two major classes of drugs are used to treat depressive disorders: the tricyclic/tetracyclic antidepressants and the monoamine oxidase inhibitors. The latter require following a special diet because they interact with tryamine, which is found in cheeses, beer, wine, chicken livers, and other foods, and causes elevation of blood pressure. The tricyclic antidepressants require no special diet; common generic drugs in this class are amitriptyline, desipramine, doxepin, and imipramine. Lithium carbonate, a common mineral, is used to control the manic phase of manic-depressive illness. In smaller doses, it is also used to regulate the mood fluctuations of this bipolar disorder.

Today, the medical community, with some strong dissenters, considers the drug most commonly called Prozac to be a true revolution in the treatment of depression. Prozac is actually one of many drugs classified as serotonin reuptake inhibitors.

As this classification indicates, Prozac and its brethren inhibit the flow of a substance called serotonin in the brain. Medical researchers have recently found that shortly after ingestion, foods influence the release of important brain chemicals and that carbohydrate foods, in particular, trigger the release of serotonin, which, in turn, suppresses the desire for carbohydrates. Such a mechanism may have evolved to prevent people from glutting themselves on carbohydrates and failing to procure harder-to-find protein. Until recent times, carbohydrate foods were far more accessible than protein. Serotonin is believed to work in complex relationships with insulin and several amino acids, especially trypto-phan, all of which participate in monitoring the appetite for various food types. In this same area of research, nutrition experts are trying to unravel the relationship between diabetes and obesity and the role that sweets play for people with these afflic-tions.

Serotonin is found in many neurons in the brain stem; collectively, these neurons form so-called sero-toninergic pathways. Noradrenaline is found in other nerve cells, and together they make up noradrener-gic pathways. Similarly, nerve cells containing acetylcholine make up cholinergic pathways. Recent research indicates that the regulation of body tem-perature, eating behavior, and perhaps sleep depends significantly on a fine balance in the activi-ty of these chemically coded pathways.

Depression may be caused by some sort of mal-function in the production, breakdown, and cellular activity of the neurotransmitters in the limbic sys-tem. A fundamental action on the brain of a tranquil-izer or other mind-altering drug is to restore the bal-ance between two or more neurotransmitters or to otherwise alter a certain neurotransmitter system. Amino acids and hormonelike substances found in brain cells for example, peptides also are believed to play an important role in moderating the activity of nerve cells and the transmission of their impulses.

Thousands of neuroscientists throughout the world are today involved in studying these chemical systems. Human understanding of how the brain operates, from its basic physiology to its role in learning and emotion, lies in gaining knowledge of the brain's chemistry under normal and abnormal conditions.

Serotonin reuptake inhibitors are still at the forefront of the battle against depression, but at last, its star is beginning to tarnish.

For one reason, European doctors have discovered that a common herb known as St. John's Wort, is perhaps far more effective at treating depression than the super high tech and super synthetic Prozac and its cousins.

St. John's Wort (wort is the old English word for flower) is a common name for annual and perennial herbs and shrubs of the family Clusiaceae, native to subtropical and temperate regions worldwide. Some species of the widespread genus Hypericum are cultivated in garden borders and rock gardens. The plants have opposite, toothless leaves, generally dotted with blackish spots, which are oil-bearing glands.

Heretofore considered a pesky weed which American farmers have tried to eliminate, this plant may revolutionize the treatment of depression. It has already nearly drive Prozac out of the market in Germany and a couple of other European nations.

And what about pregnenolone? With Prozac and St. John's Wort already carrying on a fierce battle against the dragon of depression, does pregnenolone have anything new to offer. The answer is yes.

That's because the "miracles" of Prozac and St. John's Wort are not miracles for everyone. There is a significant segment of the population that does not respond to either of the above, so there is always room for "one more" depression treatment regime.

Pregnenolone may be the perfect "gap filler" in the modern arsenal of depression medications.

Furthermore, the decline in the natural hormone levels of the body almost invariably coincide with a certain loss of zest or interest in the daily activities of life.

In a recent study, researchers discovered that elderly people who are depressed have lower levels of pregnenolone in their cerebral spinal fluid, a fluid which engulfs the brain. Also depressed people seem to contain too much of a neurotransmitter called GABA. The function of GABA is to protect the brain from getting overheated, an important function to be sure. Problems arise, however, when the brain gets too much of a good thing. In the case of too much GABA, the brain becomes sluggish, and neuro-transmitter flow is inhibited to a degree. Pregnenolone appears to counter the thickening of

GABA, and hence, may be a treatment for depression, or a general feeling of low energy and lack of ambition or zest for life. Studies still need to be done. Pregnenolone's effect on depression is still waiting for large-scale tests to prove out the theory of its counter-effect on depression.

An Arthritis Cure?

Back in the 1950s, medical researchers were conducting experiments with pregnenolone on people with rheumatoid arthritis, and they were achieving some very promising results. The investigation petered out, however, because at about the same time, researchers discovered the seemingly miraculous effect that a class of drugs called cortisols had on arthritis.

Hydrocortisone, also known as cortisol, are common names for 17-hydroxy-corticosterone, the principal hormone secreted by the outer layer, or cortex, of the adrenal gland. Hydrocortisone affects the metabolism of carbohydrate, protein, and fat; the maturation of white blood cells; the retention of salt and water in the body; the activity of the nervous system; and the regulation of blood pressure. Secretion of hydrocortisone from the adrenal cortex is stimulated by the pituitary hormone ACTH.

Because of their widespread effects, hydrocortisone and related compounds, called corticosteroids, or corticoids, are employed for many medical purposes. They are used to treat a deficiency of adrenal cortical hormones, a condition called congenital adrenal hyperplasia, rheumatoid disease that is not helped by milder drugs, and to counter severe non-infectious inflammations. Corticosteroids suppress the immune response, so they are used to increase acceptance of transplants.

Other conditions for which they are helpful are asthma, collagen diseases, and eye inflammations. Because corticosteroids affect so many body processes, they must be used carefully. Corticosteroids dispose persons to infection and can lead to swelling of the face and limbs, muscle weakness, weight gain, high blood pressure, and diabetes.

Another naturally occurring corticosteroid hormone, called cortisone, was the first corticosteroid to be isolated in 1935. It was synthesized in 1944 and subsequently became available for widespread medical use. Cortisone is rapidly converted to hydrocortisone in the body. Synthetic corticosteroids with more specific activity have now been made and are preferred in many situations.

At first cortisone seemed a cure, but as time went on, the negative side effects of cortisone became clear. While cortisone greatly eases the pain and inflammation of arthritis and many other inflammatory conditions, it also destroys bone density, makes people highly susceptible to infections, causes weight gain, "moon face," which is a characteristic widening of the neck and face, hair loss, diabetes and more. Furthermore, when people go off cortisone, they can have a heart attack, stoke or any number of other problems. That's because once you start administering artificial cortisone to a human body, the body depresses the production of its own natural cortisone-like compounds. Remove the artificial substance, and the body is left defenseless against all manner of agonizing conditions.

Still, the major drug companies realized that cortisone was very profitable, while pregnenolone, a natural substance produced by the body, had relatively low market value. Thus, it is very difficult to find money or a drug company that will waste its time testing products for which no future profits will result from. That's why cortisone and its cousins have moved forward, while pregnenolone has been all but forgotten as a possible treatment for arthritis.

NOTES

_____

_____

_____

_____

_____

_____

_____

_____

Chapter 3

Testosterone

W hen feminist women want to take a stab at what they consider the boorish, dominant or aggressive nature of men, they sometimes use the quip: "He's got testosterone poisoning."

They are right about one thing: testosterone is the hormone most associated with maleness. An aggressive sex drive. Strength. Powerful muscles. Facial hair and chest hair. The dominance of the hormone testosterone is what makes manhood ... well, manhood!

Testosterone is the principal male hormone produced mainly in the Leydig cells in the male testes. The Leydig cells also produce two other androgens of less potency and in much smaller quantities.

Testosterone stimulates the development of the male secondary sex characteristics after puberty, causing growth of the beard and pubic hair, development of the penis, and change of voice. The hormone also aids in the growth, muscular development, and masculine body contour of the adult male.

If, before puberty, little or no testosterone secretion occurs, secondary sexual characteristics fail to develop. In addition, the long bones continue to grow abnormally and give the patient a characteristic tall but effeminate build. If testicular failure follows puberty, less obvious changes occur, although gradual recession of beard, weakening of muscles, increased deposition of fat, and change in voice may develop slowly, with infertility usually present and decreased libido and sexual potential common. The hormone is often useful in treating certain types of breast cancer in women.

In the sexually undifferentiated embryo, testosterone stimulates the development of the Wolffian duct system, the forerunner of the male genital tract. Later, testosterone, along with gonadotrophins released by the pituitary gland, stimulates spermatogenesis. The Mcllerian duct system, the forerunner of the female genital tract in the female embryo, probably differentiates spontaneously without hormonal stimulus. After female sex is well defined, estradiol, produced in the ovaries and the placenta, plays a major role in the development and the functioning of the female reproductive tract.

Elderly men who take testosterone report a remarkable return of those things that were most powerful in their youths — mainly their sex drives and physical strength. It makes men feel like they are in their prime. Testosterone improves stamina and gives energy. Like pregnenolone, it also seems to make men more optimistic and forward looking about life in general.

Testosterone gets to work quickly on the men who take it. Improvement in sex drive, strength and mood occurs in just days.

The opposite — a low testosterone level — results in a loss of interest in sex, a factor which depresses many men in and of itself. Psychologically, and perhaps for not entirely all the best reasons, men associate their sex drive with their sense of manhood and inner well-being. Lack of a sex drive makes for a moody depressed man, seemingly lacking in purpose and true interest in life. But such feelings are probably much deeper and more psychological than the way we make this sound.

As modern men raise their consciousness about who and what they are, and what their role on planet earth is, such things as how much sex they have, or don't have, or want to have take a back seat to deeper elements of the male psyche. Men are discovering that they also can be nurturing, and that their aggression, including their sexual aggression, is best channeled into constructive pursuits, rather than seeing who can "score the most."

But whether it is on some deeper level of meaning, or just a surface factor, testosterone without a doubt plays an extremely important role in how a man feels about himself both physically and psychologically.

Wilbert L., of Spokane, Washington, was 62 years old, a widower, but deeply in love with a beautiful

woman of 48 who had recently come into his life, res-
cuing him from his loneliness Wilbert and Doris
related perfectly to each other on many levels. But
the one area of their relationship that lacked zing
was the sexual aspect.

A warm and loving relationship did not seem to be
enough for Wilbert to regain his interest in sex,
which had dwindled greatly since the death of this
wife eight years ago. Up until the point he met Doris,
Wilbert assumed it was depression over the loss of
his wife that had killed his once vigorous sex drive.
But he had long ago come to terms with the death of
his wife, and now here was Doris, an extremely beautiful woman of 48 who looked 35, and who still maintained a strong interest in sex.

Wilbert's lack of interest was a definite stumbling
block in an otherwise wonderful relationship.
Wilbert knew that sooner or later, Doris would inter-
pret the sexual coldness as lack of interest.
Eventually, their relationship would become like a
caring "brother-sister" arrangement, but nothing more.

During Wilbert's annual check-up, he shared with
his doctor a concern about his possible impotence.
Finding him otherwise in good physical health,
Wilbert's doctor decided to take a look at his
patient's testosterone level. Sure enough, it was low.
The doctor asked Wilbert if he would like to try
testosterone therapy. He told Wilbert that he was
not necessarily impotent, just a bit low on the substance that stimulates a healthy sex drive.

Feeling he had nothing to loose, Wilbert agreed.
Within two days of the application of a testosterone

skin patch, Wilbert's sex drive roared back to life. Almost overnight, Wilbert felt like a sex-starved teenager and simply couldn't wait to whisk Doris away for a romantic weekend in some secluded location where they could have plenty of time for ... well, let's just call it intimacy. Their relationship was saved, not just because sex was added to it, but because all good relationship are made up of a balance of things, including shared values, similarities in likes and dislikes, compatible spiritual beliefs and more. Remove any one of these major elements and a relationship can crumble like a house of cards. Good relationships are only as strong as their weakest links. If one of those links is a stone cold sex life, the relationship may be doomed to failure.

There is a pervasive belief that the older people get, the more their sex drive goes down. This is an absolute myth, however. Most healthy people of advanced age report that they continue to have sex on a regular basis, if not as frequently, but with more quality and satisfaction.

There is no reason for senior citizens to simply accept the fact that a loss of their sex drive is a natural aspect of growing old. Testosterone, DHEA, estrogen and melatonin replacement therapy can play an important role in ensuring that a normal sex drive does not shrink away to nothing as the years roll by.

Testosterone not only ensures a healthy sex drive in aging men, but also maintain strong muscle tone, a high energy level and a clear-headed, positive outlook on life. The number of men who are currently taking testosterone supplements number in the hundreds of thousands, and most medical observers agree that there will soon be as many men taking testosterone as there are women taking estrogen supplements.

There is case study after case study to prove that testosterone therapy works for aging men. Every day, doctors see before their very eyes the living proof that much of what we all have long believed about the aging process no longer holds true. Loss of sex drive, loss of muscle tone, loss of that feeling of youthful vigor, and even the loss of hair and smooth skin need not ravish men as they move past 50 and into their senior years of 70, 80 and 90. In fact, age 75 should be the beginning of a new term in the lives of men that ideally could last another 40 to 50 years.

More good news about testosterone is the fact that is is now easier to administer than ever before. Thank "the patch" for that. Recently approved by the FDA, a patch containing testosterone which is applied to the skin replaced the old method for delivering testosterone to the body, which was either injection, or a patch worn directly on the scrotum — hardly an appealing idea to most men. The new testosterone patches can be worn on the arm or the back, are painless and hardly noticeable at all, except for the fantastic effect it has on recharging and restoring youth to thousands of men who had given up hope on their long lost younger years.

Adding testosterone to the blood of aging men makes as much sense as adding estrogen to menopausal women. Doctors are now coming to believe that just as women find their natural hormone production disrupted at the point of menopause, men too have a time clocking ticking inside them which eventually tells the body: "It's time to wind down and grow old now!"

Sometimes called "male menopause", this sudden decline in the general health and virility of the male physical body is the result of reduced testosterone, just as female menopause is the result of a turn down in estrogen production. Perhaps the problem with male menopause is the fact that there is no clear point of distinction for onset of this condition as there is in women. For women, the loss of the period, the shedding of the last egg, is a clear, easily recognized "event" that takes place in such a way that can be marked on a calender. A woman can say: "It was in the fall of 1995 that I stopped menstruating and entered menopause." But a man has no such definite way to measure his turning point. Aging effects sneak up on him gradually, and when they do, it is most often accepted as "natural", and little is done about it.

But if women are so readily prescribed the female hormone estrogen at a certain time in their lives, why not do the same for men, and prescribe the male hormone testosterone?

Once again, we should mention that not all men experience a decline in their testosterone levels. Many men obviously stay vigorous and healthy naturally late into their senior years. Only about 30 percent of men actually experience a significant drop in their testosterone, and thus "qualify" for the benefits of testosterone therapy. But the 30 percent that does see a decline in natural testosterone production represent millions of men, and these men should have some kind of viable alternative to what genetics and Mother Nature has doled out for them.

Johns Hopkins' scientists studying testosterone-replacement therapy report that the primary male sex hormone may affect some learning skills, including improving visual and perceptual abilities. The findings may provide additional insight into testosterone's role in the brain.

"This is an interesting, early finding and it highlights the importance of studying the effects of sex hormones on brain function," says Adrian Dobs, M.D., senior author and an associate professor of medicine.

Results of the study, funded by the National Institutes of Health, were presented June 14 at the International Congress of Endocrinology's annual meeting in San Francisco. Ten men with low testosterone underwent word, memory, coordination and other learning tests while on and off testosterone treatment. When receiving testosterone, they had improved visual and spatial skills and a better "mental grasp of objects" — fitting building blocks into the correct spaces, identifying pictures and remembering shapes, patterns and locations- the results showed. When not receiving testosterone, the men showed improved verbal fluency and verbal memory — making up sentences, defining words and recalling words from a test.

Researchers at Hopkins and elsewhere are studying whether testosterone-replacement therapy may improve men's muscle mass and strength, bone density, cholesterol level, sense of well-being, cognitive function and balance.

"Compared to estrogen research, we're 15 years behind in investigating the benefits of testosterone," says Dobs.

Testosterone replacement therapy has been shown to improve sexual function in men with low testosterone, while many studies suggest that estrogen replacement therapy reduces the risk of heart disease and osteoporosis in women after menopause.

Testosterone, like many other hormones, is produced only at certain sites in the body. It does very limited, specific functions and is quickly metabolized. When testosterone was found to build muscle tissue and to cause the development of male secondary sex characteristics, medical researchers tried to use testosterone to treat diseases that caused the loss of muscle mass.

Unfortunately, testosterone in its natural form has a half life of only about ten minutes in the body. This means that half of the dose of testosterone is metabolized away in as little as ten minutes after it is absorbed. Half of what remains is broken down every ten minutes after that. At the end of an hour, none of the original dose of testosterone can be detected in the body. Injecting natural testosterone into muscle can make it last as long as ten hours, but this is still not nearly long enough to be useful as a medicine.

Medicinal chemists began to alter natural testosterone in an attempt to make drugs that would work like testosterone but last long enough in the body to have an effect. After extensive testing, they found that changing the testosterone molecule at one of only a few specific places would give them what they wanted—anabolic steroid drugs. These variations are known by chemists as "17-alpha-alkylates," "17-beta-esters" and "1-methyle steroids." All anabolic steroids in use today are variations of one of those three changes to the testosterone molecule. These chemical classes of anabolics are taken by different routes and have different side effects on the body. The 17-alpha-alkylates and 1-methyl compounds are taken by mouth, while 17-beta-esters must be injected to be effective. For convenience, they will be classified here as oral or injectable steroids.

Testosterone in Women

Although testosterone is considered the "male hormone," the fact is, women produce testosterone too. The difference between men and women is that in men, testosterone is dominant, and in women, estrogen is dominant. Yet, males and females need both hormones to survive. That begs the medical question: Should a sexually dysfunctional woman be prescribed testosterone? Experts are quick to take sides.

In _**The Hormone of Desire: The Truth About Sexuality, Menopause, and Testosterone**_, psychiatrist Susan Rako writes that women lose much of their testosterone, as well as estrogen, at menopause. A very low testosterone level interferes with a woman's sex drive.

But many experts say prescribing testosterone for women is untested. Although there is currently "a big sell going on for testosterone," there are no long-term studies to back up its use, says Dr. Wulf Utian of the University Hospitals of Cleveland. "You want the same kind of scrutiny we had for hormone replacement therapy."

Says Dr. Sadja Greenwood of the University of California Medical School: "Women should not be told testosterone is the hormone of desire. . . . So many times women have been given medications before the long-term consequences are in. Is this another case?"

Salt Lake City endocrinologist Dr. Kirtly Parker Jones says: "Women now think they can take this hormone to make them more interested in sex. A woman's interest in sex is 95% psychological and about 5% physiological. This issue has been very sensationalized."

But testosterone has its champions. Dr. Barbara Bartlik, Cornell University Medical College, says: "We could work with women in sex therapy, treat their depression, but we still could not fix their sexual responsiveness unless we first fix their testosterone levels."

Manhattan reproductive endocrinologist Dr. Hugh Melnick says of possible side effects such as facial hair: "Women won't become masculinized on low doses of testosterone. Each woman's treatment program is individualized."

More on Testosterone and Sex Drive

Just about any man who remembers his teen age years also remembers that sex was just about all he could think about most of the time. And 18-year-old male certainly has "sex on the brain," with studies showing that the average teen age male actually thinks about sex at least once every five minutes!

As a man ages, that figure goes down to about once every 15 minutes. That's still a lot, yet it represents a 30 percent decline in general interest in sex. As a man ages even further, when he tips 50 and goes beyond, the sex drive tends to dwindle further.

Still, it is important to note that is it dangerous to oversimplify this issue of male sexuality. The frequency of desire for sex, or even the frequency of the sex act itself is not the only measure, and perhaps not even the best measure of a normal and healthy sex life for the average man.

The older a man gets, the more he realizes that it is not how much sex he has, but the quality of the sex he has. Many men have some confusion about this. Men invariably get trapped in peer pressure situations and distorted media images of what "normal" sexual desire and behavior is. But the facts are that there is no "normal" sexual behavior. Just as each man is an individual, the interest or lack of interest in sex varies from man to man. For some men, sex once a month is the optimum amount of sex, while others simply "must" have sex every day.

For the man who is accustomed to having sex every day, a sudden slow down in sexual desire or ability to perform can be much more traumatic than a man who has sex only once a month. For the second man, a slow down in sex drive may not become apparent for several months, and even then, the loss would not be as critical because sex was only an infrequent activity in the first place.

Still, men who lose their testosterone levels should be considered a class all to themselves. Lack of proper testosterone amounts means a man no longer has a choice about when or how often he wants to have sex. Lack of a sustained sex drive can have far reaching effects on the life of a man or woman. Maintaining long-term relationships become especially problematic since sex is such an integral part of a human relationship.

Men with dwindling testosterone levels not only have less interest in sex, but the actual sex they do have will be less enjoyable. They may have trouble getting an erection. They may be unable to ejaculate. The entire sensory experience of sex will be dulled, less exciting and less pleasurable. **Because so many men are taught to hide their feelings, and to cover up any perceived self-inadequacies, a dropped testosterone level can lead to a kind of "cover up mentality." Here's an example:**

Gene K., a university professor, was 55 years old and during the past year, he noticed his interest in sex all but disappeared. An intelligent, well-educated man, Gene suspected he may have a medical problem, but he was also afraid that his sudden loss of interest in sex was "all in his head." Like most men, Gene would only go to a doctor as a last resort. After all, he had never been sick a day in his life. He had little use for doctors for most of his life, and he was not about to go scampering to one now. Additionally, the idea of the embarrassment of explaining the fact that he just didn't have interest in sex anymore was not something he was psychologically comfortable with.

The trouble is, Gene's wife, Karen, had no idea what was going on in her husband's mind or body. Why the sudden lack of interest in sex? Was he losing interest in her? Was he having an affair with another woman? Was he turning gay? Was he sick?

Rather than discussing his problem openly and honestly with his wife, Gene just pushed her away. He became more distant, not because he wanted to be, but simply because he could not admit that his sex drive was nowhere. When Karen would make sexual overtures, he found a convenient way to duck away or change the subject. Of course, it didn't take long for Karen to become confused, angry and afraid that their 25-year marriage was coming to a slow halt.

Still, Gene and Karen had a strong love. Gene knew that he would have to confront his issue of drooping sexuality or loose the love of his life. Finally, he agreed to undergo marriage counseling. In the course of the their sessions with a qualified marriage counselor, the therapist quickly concluded that Gene and Karen had an extremely strong marriage. They were on the same page on just about every issue and always had been, except for this past year of Gene's sudden and strange lack of interest in bedroom activity. Using logical deduction, the therapist zeroed in on Gene sex drive — or lack of it — as the primary problem.

Before going further with "talk therapy" the marriage counselor suggested Gene get a physical examination, including a test of his blood. The therapist suspected that, like so many men in their mid-50s, Gene may have been experiencing a drop in his testosterone level.

To Gene's utter and complete surprise, that was exactly the case. Gene's problem was not in his head, and the problem was not that he did not love his wife. The problem was in his blood chemistry.

Now, just a few years ago, a doctor noticing depleted testosterone levels in Gene's blood might have said: "Well, it's to be expected. Aging men inevitably lose their sex drives. It's time to take up a new hobby — sailing perhaps?"

But Gene's doctor refused to take that attitude. No longer should a depleted testosterone level be thought of as normal, any more than a low white blood cell count should be thought of as normal. If Gene's blood test would have indicated he was low on iron, or high on cholesterol, the doctor would certainly prescribe medication or a special diet to bring these factors back into balance. So why not bring the testosterone level back into proper balance?

Gene's doctor applied a prescribed a testosterone skin patch, and within two days, Gene's sex drive had returned — just like that.

Gene and his wife not only made love for the first time in many months — they went away for a romantic weekend in a beautiful resort area, but took in none of the sights. Gene said they did nothing but make love for three days straight. They barely set foot outside the bedroom for the entire trip!

Better than his sex drive, Gene's marriage was back on track. Both he and Karen were enormously relieved that there wasn't something deeper and more permanently wrong with their wonderful marriage. For want of a few milligrams of a natural body chemical, testosterone, Gene and Karen may have ended up as just another statistic in the pages of divorce court records.

Please keep in mind that not all cases of sexual problems are as easily solved as Gene's was. The human sexual mechanism is highly complex, and a lot can go wrong. Problems are not always clear cut, and often can combine both psychological and physical factors. For example, such common diseases as diabetes and atherosclerosis can impair blood flow to the penis, making it difficult for a man to get an erection and experience sexual stimulation. In these latter two cases, testosterone therapy will probably be of little direct help ... on the other hand, there may be some kind of connection that is still too complex to be understood.

Much more research needs to be done. In fact, the whole field of male sexual performance has not exactly been one of high priority for the medical community, even though significant advances have been made. The full role of testosterone on male sexuality is a book that has yet to be written, but the promise of many new and exciting advances is great.

Can Testosterone Aid in Depression?

A man in a bad mood is generally not a man who wants to have sex. A man who does not have a lot of sex is generally in a bad mood.

What we are trying to say here is that a healthy sex drive contributes to a positive attitude in most men. For good or bad, the majority of men still peg their manhood on their sexual prowess, whether it be with their own wives, or out there "playing the field." A dangerous thing to do in this day of AIDS and other sexually transmitted diseases.

But the **"good sex/good mood"** may have connection that go deeper than psychology. Is the body chemistry that makes for good sex associated with the same mixture that makes for a good mood?

There is a lot of anecdotal evidence that testosterone not only boosts the sex drive, but generally makes men happier and gives them a general feeling of joy and good mood.

In one double blind study, a group of men were given testosterone for three months and a placebo for another three months. Neither the subject nor the researcher knew when they received the testosterone, and when the received the "blanks." After a three-month period, the men were asked to correctly name the months they received the real thing, and those when they did not. All but one of the men answered correctly on all counts. Some 98% of the men were able to tell the difference between real testosterone in their blood and lower levels.

They reported stronger sex drives, more aggressiveness and certainty in their business dealings, and a general, higher sense of well-being. While American doctors still do not prescribe testosterone for mild depression in men over the age of 50, British doctors have been doing so for several years and with great success. In Britain, there is a general feeling that men undergo a hormone crisis similar to that of women undergoing menopause and rapid reductions in their estrogen levels.

Not all of the men need to stay on testosterone for long periods. Sometimes just a few months brings many men back to feeling like their "old self." More recently, some doctors are switching men to DHEA after an initial round of testosterone therapy. That's because DHEA is converted into testosterone by the body. After a man gets back on his feet, DHEA can help him stay there after testosterone treatment is finished.

Testosterone as Energy Booster

Men who take testosterone almost unanimously report a surge in their physical strength and energy. Almost all of them use the term "youthful" when they describe this welcome new condition. To understand how testosterone can boost energy and muscle strength, one must look to the physiology of blood and muscle.

Sports doctors recognize two kinds of exercise: isotonic and isometric. Isotonic exercise involves moving a muscle through a long distance against low resistance, as in running, swimming, or gymnastics. In isometric exercise, on the other hand, muscles are moved through a short distance against a high resistance, as in pushing or pulling an immovable object. Isometric exercise is best for developing large muscles, whereas isotonic exercise has beneficial effects on the cardiovascular system. It increases the amount of blood that the heart can pump and causes proliferation of small blood vessels that carry oxygen to the muscles.

These changes make possible longer sustained activity. Neither kind of exercise increases the number of muscle fibers, but both types, and especially isometric exercise, increase the thickness of the muscle fibers and their ability to store glycogen, the fuel for muscular activity.

The most common respiratory pigment is hemoglobin, which is present in the blood of most mammals and consists of an iron compound of hematin combined with a globulin. In certain insects the blood pigment is hemocyanin, a compound similar to hemoglobin, in which the iron is replaced by copper. The most important property of the respiratory pigments is an affinity for oxygen. The pigment forms a loose chemical combination with oxygen when exposed to an atmosphere rich in that element, as in the capillaries of respiratory organs such as gills or lungs. The oxygen compound is more acidic than the pigment and consequently absorbs sodium ions from the sodium carbonate-bicarbonate solution in the blood plasma, forcing the latter to release carbon dioxide. When the blood reaches the tissues, the oxygen balance is reversed; the blood pigment releases oxygen and, becoming more basic, also releases sodium ions, which combine with the carbon dioxide from the tissues to form sodium bicarbonate. The interchange of gases in the blood is called external respiration; that taking place in the body, between the blood and tissues, is called internal respiration.

Red blood cells carry oxygen to all part of the human body. Men who take testosterone see their red blood cell count rise. Thus, they get more oxygen from brain to the muscles in their toes. The end result is every muscle and every organ in the body being energized. The man not only feels more clear headed because his brain is getting more oxygen, but his muscles and organs have more fuel to perform their tasks with, and they operate at a higher level of efficiency.

Closely associated to all this is "getting flabby." We're talking about loss of muscle tone with age, and the actual loss of muscle tissue itself, along with a gain in body fat. Most medical researchers find this process is directly related to dwindling rates of testosterone in aging men.

But once again, why should we accept this as "natural." We do not accept other harmful changes in the blood chemistry as natural. A man low in vitamin C can develop the disease of scurvy. A man low in iron can become anemic. A man low in vitamin D can suffer from bone thinning and an increase in broken bones. In all cases, doctors would readily consider these conditions as "deficiencies," and would prescribe supplements to make up for them. Why not then take the same tact with testosterone? No, we should not accept a shrinking testosterone level and all it entails — lower sex drive, loss of muscle tissue and tone, depression and more — as natural. Not when it all can easily be reversed with a testosterone patch.

Why are doctors still hesitant to prescribe testosterone. One reason is the possibility of prostate enlargement and cancer, which testosterone may indeed be involved in. On the other hand, men who have a clean bill of health, and who already have unnaturally low levels should experience no harm in bringing their levels back up to the level to which they had previously been throughout their lives, especially their youthful years.

In 1996, the highly respected "New England Journal of Medicine" reported that testosterone can increase the muscle mass in men and women by a significant degree, and that it can do so even without exercise. Another study showed that testosterone injections for in elderly men increased both their muscle mass and their strength.

It should be noted that adding testosterone to the blood mixture of men may cause them to become more active, and perhaps take up more physical activity, such as swimming, bike riding, jogging, tennis or any one of a number of enjoyable pastimes. This in turn would have the effect of increasing muscle tone and mass and reducing fat.

So we see that testosterone not only biochemically and physiologically builds the body, but is also creates the mental attitude and energy level that makes men more likely to treat their bodies like they should be treated. Low testosterone levels do the opposite. A man who has no energy at the end of a long day at the office is much more likely to crash in front of the TV with a six-pack of beer or a half-dozen donuts than suit up and head out for an invigorating five-mile run.

And this brings up another important point: testosterone therapy, and any kind of hormone therapy for that matter, should not be considered a "blank check" and substitute for treating your body well. If you smoke tobacco products, drink a lot of alcohol, have a lousy high fat, high sodium, high sugar diet, even the most fortified and resistant body can succumb to illnesses of all kinds. Testosterone, DHEA, pregnenolone and all the rest are not magic wands giving us immunity to whatever punishment we hand out to our poor physical bodies.

Testosterone and Alzheimer's Disease

Since the entire topic of this book concerns staying young, we would be remiss if we did not discuss one of the most prominent diseases that robs human beings of their youth — Alzheimer's Disease.

Alzheimer's Disease is a progressive degenerative disease of the brain now considered a leading cause of dementia. First described by the German neuropathologist Alois Alzheimer (1864-1915) in 1906, it affects an estimated 2.5 to 3 million persons in the U.S. The incidence of the disease increases with advancing age, but there is no evidence that it is caused by the aging process.

The average life expectancy of persons with the disease is between five and ten years, although many patients now survive 15 years or more due to improvements in care and medical treatment. The cause of this disease has not been discovered, although palliative therapy is available. The ability of doctors to diagnose Alzheimer's disease has improved over the last ten years, but this remains a process of elimination and final diagnosis can be confirmed only at autopsy.

At autopsy, Alzheimer's patients show nerve cell loss in the parts of the brain associated with cognitive functioning. The hallmark lesions of Alzheimer's disease include the formation of abnormal proteins known as neurofibrillary tangles and neuritic plaques. The nature of these abnormal proteins and the location of the gene for producing the precursor protein has been identified. Alzheimer's disease is also characterized by profound deficits in the brain's neurotransmitters, chemicals that transmit nerve impulses, particularly acetylcholine, which has been linked with memory function. The important scientific issue concerning Alzheimer's disease revolves around the question of why particular classes of nerve cells are vulnerable and subject to cell death. Many researchers are actively pursuing an answer to this question in studies examining the potential effects of genetic factors, toxins, infectious agents, metabolic abnormalities, and a combination of these factors. Recent findings indicate that a small percentage of Alzheimer's cases may be inherited.

But now new research is indicating that hormones may play a vital role in causing or preventing this dreaded disease.

Doctors have already observed that women who take estrogen after menopause have smaller incidence of the disease. They believe testosterone can have the same positive effect in men. Much of the reason for believing so comes from studies with mice. In a number of tests with aging and artificially aged mice, testosterone injections and implants proved to prevent a significant amount of mice from developing senile dementia. At this point there is not enough data of elderly men who have taken testosterone supplements consistently and long enough to make accurate measures of how well it may reduce the incidence of AD in men. Because of the large number of women who are put on estrogen supplements for purposes of treating post menopausal disorders, there is more data available as to how the female hormone, estrogen, apparently prevents a significant percentage of women from contracting AD.

Testosterone and the Human Brain

Understanding how testosterone makes the brain work better will be better understood if we first take a brief look at the biochemistry of the brain.

Metabolic processes in the brain depend on a steady supply of glucose and oxygen carried by the blood by means of the arteries. Nerve cells require both substances in abundant amounts because of their constant physiological activity, day and night. Many substances circulating in the blood do not enter the brain because tiny elements — in both the choroid plexus of the ventricles and the capillary beds within the brain — act as a molecular and ionic filter. This filtration system is called the blood-brain barrier. Many biological compounds having a high molecular weight, such as adrenal hormones or amino acids, do not pass through this barrier readily, and certain smaller molecules and even ions do not penetrate the barrier at all, because of their ionic charge. Thus, the chemistry of the brain is kept in equilibrium and well protected from the abnormal chemical challenges often posed by what humans eat and drink.

The nerve or glial cells in different areas of the brain are classified not only by their starlike anatomical shape but also by their chemical makeup. Individual neurons contain one of many different neurotransmitters that are used for communication from one cell to another. For example, the neurohormone serotonin is found in many neurons in the brain stem; collectively, these neurons form so-called serotoninergic pathways. Noradrenaline is found in other nerve cells, and together they make up noradrenergic pathways. Similarly, nerve cells containing acetylcholine make up cholinergic pathways. Recent research indicates that the regulation of body temperature, eating behavior, and perhaps sleep depends significantly on a fine balance in the activity of these chemically coded pathways.

Certain psychiatric states may also be caused by some sort of malfunction in the production, breakdown, and cellular activity of the neurotransmitters in the limbic system. A fundamental action on the brain of a tranquilizer or other mind-altering drug is to restore the balance between two or more neurotransmitters or to otherwise alter a certain neurotransmitter system. Amino acids and hormonelike substances found in brain cells for example, peptides also are believed to play an important role in moderating the activity of nerve cells and the transmission of their impulses.

Human understanding of how the brain operates, from its basic physiology to its role in learning and emotion, lies in gaining knowledge of the brain's chemistry under normal and abnormal conditions.

A key way that testosterone helps the brain is by increasing the red blood cell count in the blood stream. Because the brain is vitally dependent on glucose and on oxygen, it needs a rigorous and healthy supply of both, and both are supplied by red blood cells. In men who are experiencing dwindling testosterone levels, it is small wonder that they feel less clear headed, more tired, "cloudy" and forgetful. Their brains simply are not getting the basic ingredients they need to function at peak levels.

In the hippocampus of the brain, a hormone called a LH-RH is produced. This stands for luteinizing hormone-releasing hormone. This is the substance that stimulates the pituitary gland to produce LH, which then stimulates the testes to manufacture testosterone. But as men age, levels of testosterone

production fall off. Cells then receive less LH receptors. These receptors are needed for LH to attach
itself to.

What this adds up to is that the testes are losing
communication with the pituitary glands.
Significantly, and at the same time, there is an
increase in the number of LH-RH receptors back in
the hippocampus, which is a clear indication that
the brain is trying to make up for the loss of receptors on the testes. The brain and the testes are
working at odds with each other. The brain is trying
to increase testosterone production while the testes
are trying to slow the whole process down. The
testes usually win this battle of will and the brain
gives up on the whole process.

The fact that the testes will no longer "do their
job" is yet another argument for testosterone supplements, which will compensate for this brain-
testes conflict, which is common in most older men.

Testosterone and the Heart

Young men almost never die of heart disease, but
when they grow over the age of 45 to 50, heart disease become the No. 1 killer of men. **Why?**

Why are young men almost immune to heart problems and older men dying from them by the hundreds of thousands? Well, it doesn't take a rocket
scientist to see a connection between aging and
problems with the heart. And if the effects of aging
could be slowed safely and effectively with a simple
supplement of a readily available hormone, should-
n't this be done? We believe so.

When you consider the fact that more than 90,000 men die every year, doing something to counter heart disease becomes more than a good idea, but a moral imperative.

Testosterone has long been known and used in Europe as a remedy for a wide variety of problems which produce heart disease, including poor circulation, clogged arteries, diabetes, obesity, high cholesterol and more.

If doctor's in Europe have been successfully treating thousands of cases of heart disease with testosterone, why isn't the same approach used in the United States?

The most likely answer is medical politics and economics. Open heart surgery is one of the most expensive and prestigious fields for a modern physician to be involved in. Heart surgery is a major money maker for hospitals and clinics and a career enhancer for doctors who like the superstar adulation normally reserved for actors or popular politicians.

Is surgery more effective than alternative treatments? Surprisingly, the answer may be no. Recent studies have shown that men who undergo open heart surgery don't necessarily live longer, or see a significant improvement in their health than do those who do not have the operation.

Does open heart surgery help some people and save lives? The answer is absolutely yes, but only not as often as the medical establishment would have us believe.

Furthermore, until recently very little emphasis has been given to preventing heart disease from happening in the first place. For many years, a "holistic" approach to human health has been an absolute dirty word to the mainstream medical establishment. A holistic approach simply means taking care of the entire body so that individual parts of it stay healthy as well, including the heart.

Men should adopt a healthy, low-fat diet, and avoid all the major heart damaging habits that so many men love, including smoking, drinking, watching too much TV while munching on fat-soaked potato chips and swilling beer rather than getting outside for fresh air and exercise. If all men reformed their diets and abstained from bad habits, heart disease would be reduced to an enormous degree.

Rather than lulling men into a false sense of security which tells them: "Go ahead, live it up. We'll clean your slate later on in life with a little open heart surgery. You'll be good as new after that."

But the fact is, open heart surgery rarely returns men to their previous level of 100 percent physical capacity. Men who undergo heart surgery tire easily, are short of breath, and must limit what physical activities they want to do.

Of course, telling men NOT to do all the bad things and TO do all the good things is a bit like a priest or a minister telling his flock to never sin. We all know that is never going to happen. We are all imperfect, and most of us are going go for that sizzling steak and deliciously greasy pizza a lot more often than our internal editor wants us to.

So the second part of an answer which forms an alternative to open heart surgery is making the heart and body more resistant to all the bad things we throw at our bodies and the toll Father Time doles out.

By the way, men are not the only sex to suffer from heart disease. Women do as well, it's just that their high risk for heart disease does not start until they reach their 60s or 70s, while men start their high risk time at about age 45. Why the difference? Well, the answer is significant because the answer points to hormone depletion as the cause of heart disease.

Men see a decline in their testosterone levels usually beginning in their mid-40s to 50s. Women don't see their estrogen levels drop until after menopause, which comes nearer the 60-year mark. Also, many women who experience menopause earlier are often prescribed estrogen replacement therapy. The bottom line is, women do not have to do without optimum levels of their female hormone as much and as long as men have to do without their's.

If heart disease is greatly reduced in women who are taking estrogen supplements, it stands to reason that men taking testosterone supplements can enjoy the same benefits — namely, the reduction in incidence of heart disease.

Amazingly, for many years, the medical community generally believed that it was robust "manly men" who were most likely to have heart attacks, and that slimmer, more effeminant men were less likely to have heart attacks. The logic, we suppose, is that because women have fewer heart attacks, those men who are more like women are less likely to have heart attacks as well. But as it turns out, just the opposite is probably the case!

Women are protected from heart attacks because they have more of what makes them women — the female hormone estrogen. But men are protected from heart attacks by what makes them men — the male hormone testosterone!

Recent research seems to bare this out. In one study, a group of elderly men were examined and their testosterone levels were compared with their incidence of heart problems, such as atherosclerosis, damage to muscles, cholesterol levels and other factors, and it was found that the men with the highest cholesterol levels generally had healthier hearts and less of those conditions associated with heart problems.

It seems clear that testosterone is good for the heart, and good for men ages 45 and over. From the brain and the heart, to a man's mood and sexual performance, testosterone plays an extremely vital role in not only preventing disease, but keeping a man youthful and vigorous, and full of positive zest for life.

The medical establishment needs to take a more serious look at the promise of testosterone replacement therapy in men who experience a lowering of their male hormone level as they grow older. Maintaining the level of this hormone (and the others we will discuss in coming chapters) may mean that men will grow older — but without aging! There is no reason why a man cannot maintain a healthy muscular body with a strong heart, a robust sex drive, a positive mood and healthy aggressiveness well into his senior years, perhaps even to ages exceeding 110, 120 or beyond.

NOTES

_____

_____

_____

_____

_____

_____

_____

_____

_____

_____

Chapter 4

Estrogen

Unlike all the other ground-breaking informa-tion that is only recently coming to light about such super hormones as DHEA, melatonin, pregnenolone and the others, estrogen has been a hormone doctors have only been more than happy to prescribe to millions of women over the past 40 or 50 years.

"People always ask me in disbelief: Why on earth do you take estrogen? You look like the last person in the world who needs it! You look so young! And to that I answer: Well, why do you think I look so young! Yes, I'm 57 and it might sound like bragging to admit that I don't look a day over 38, but it's a fact.

My husband is 40, and everyone assumes I'm a year or two his junior! I've been taking estrogen for 14 years, and it's the best thing I have ever done for myself. Don't let your actual age fool you. It's just a number. Your body and mind tell the real story about whether you are young or old, and I certainly know which I am."

— Nancy G., age 51, Oak Park, IL,
one of some 10-12 million American
women currently taking estrogen.

At first, estrogen was only given to women after they received hysterectomies or developed considerable problems as the result of menopause. It wasn't long, however, that doctors noticed women on estrogen as a rule age a lot more gracefully than woman deprived of their youthful level of female hormone.

All the anecdotal evidence about the benefits spawned a large number of studies of women on estrogen therapy, and in study after study, researchers found that estrogen was the closest thing to the fountain of youth yet discovered for womankind.

Consider the following medical facts:

• Women taking estrogen do not suffer bone thinning and osteoporosis with anything near the frequency of nonestrogen users. A plague for most elderly women, estrogen reinforced women's escape from this crippling ailment.

• Estrogen-taking women had rates of heart disease more than 50 percent lower than that of nonestrogen users.

• A recent prestigious and large scale study revealed that women who take estrogen long after menopause cut their risk of developing Alzheimer's by 54 percent.

• Of the 45 percent of 472 women in the study who had taken estrogen orally or through skin patches, only nine developed Alzheimer's. Of those who did not take estrogen, 25 developed the disease.

• This study took place over a period of 16 years and was done by John Hopkins Medical Institutions, and the National Institute of Aging.

• Rates of colon cancer were vastly reduced in women taking estrogen.

Is all the news about estrogen good. No. To be honest, estrogen has been linked to increases in endometrial and breast cancer, but the actual rates of these are extremely low, and most medical researchers agree that the risk-trade off is well worth it for the majority of women.

A study which started in 1976 and which looked at 121,700 female registered nurses, found that those who took estrogen treatments cut their risk of death by 37 percent compared to those who did not. The beneficial effects seem to fall off after about 10 years, but estrogen users of more than 10 years still were 20 percent less likely to die after a decade of hormone use.

The risks also varied depending on a woman's health problems.

Those who had several risk factors for heart disease because they suffered from high blood pressure, were obese or smoked saw a 49 percent drop in their death rate if they took hormones, while women who were at low risk for heart disease had only a 13 percent decline in their likelihood of death.

When they examined specific causes of death, researchers found that hormones protected the heart even if the medicine was taken for longer than 10 years. However, after 10 years the death rate for breast cancer was 43 percent higher than it should have been.

Researchers concluded, then, that additional use of estrogen is probably offset, at least in part, by the risk of breast cancer. Still, they also concluded that the survival benefits of extended estrogen therapy outweigh the risk, but the risks and benefits vary depending on existing risk factors and the duration of hormone use and must be carefully considered by each woman.

Still, many primary medical researchers agree that the breast cancer risk should be considered minor, even though it is a reason for concern.

That's because researchers observed that the average woman's risk of death from the ages of 50 to 94 years has been estimated to be 31 percent from coronary heart disease, 2.8 percent from breast cancer, and 2.8 percent from hip fracture. The benefits of estrogen use appear to far outweigh the risks For women with a low risk of heart disease, however, the benefits of hormone therapy may not outweigh the risks.

In California, researchers studied women who started using estrogen in 1969 and have continued to do so over the past three decades. The women were born between 1900 and 1925, so all of them were already elderly or "old" when they began estrogen therapy. Compared to other women of the same age group, the death rate of the estrogen-taking women was about half as great as that of nonestrogen takers, or about 46 percent less. If you had a 46 percent less chance of dying over the next 30 years, would you take it? At any rate, all of the above studies clearly indicate that estrogen improves a woman's chance of living longer and healthier.

All fine statistics to be sure, but what a lot of researchers also fail to mention is that estrogen greatly improves the daily quality of life for most of the women who supplement their system with it, if their levels have become depleted through menopause and age. The women feel younger, they have higher levels of energy, have less body fat, greater muscle tone and their sex lives are far more stimulating and exciting than those women who are low in estrogen .

Furthermore, researchers are finding new ways to use estrogen in ways that may reduce the small risks of doing so even more. Estrogen is not administered today the same way it was just 20 or 30 years ago. The risk of uterine cancer, for example, has been all but eliminated by adding progesterone to the intake of estrogen. Progesterone stimulates periodic bleeding in postmenopausal women, sort of giving them back their periods, and thus the benefits of their periods, namely, the release of potentially cancerous tissue build-up in the uterus.

Before we look more at the exciting possibilities of estrogen and the youth renewal revolution among women it is generating, it will be helpful here to take a quick step back and examine just what estrogen is and how it fits into the greater context of the body's hormone system,

Estrogens are any of a group of female sex hormones that stimulate the appearance of secondary female sex characteristics in girls at puberty. They control growth of the lining of the uterus during the first part of the menstrual cycle, cause changes in the breasts during pregnancy, and regulate various metabolic processes. Among the better known estrogens are estrone, estradiol, and estriol, all produced primarily in the ovaries. Stilbestrol and estradiol, two synthetic estrogens, are respectively five and ten times as potent as estrone; although not related to natural estrogens, their activity is similar.

They are used to treat various conditions, including estrogen deficiencies in women (most commonly after menopause) and inflammation of the vagina. They may be used to stimulate lactation following childbirth and in the treatment, but not cure, of breast cancer in women and of advanced and even disseminated cancer of the prostate gland in men.

Estrogen is among the known hormones which belong to three chemical groups, proteins, steroids, and amines. Those in the protein, or polypeptide, group include the hormones produced by the anterior pituitary, parathyroid, placenta, and pancreas. In the steroid group are the hormones of the adrenal cortex and gonads. The amines are produced by the adrenal medulla and thyroid. The synthesis of hormones occurs intracellularly, and in most instances the product is retained within the cell until its release into the blood. The thyroid and the ovaries, however, contain special sacs for hormone storage.

Release of hormones depends on the levels in the blood of other hormones and of certain metabolic products under hormone influence, and also on nervous stimulation. The production of the anterior pituitary hormone is inhibited when the hormones produced by the particular target gland, the adrenal cortex, the thyroid, or the gonads, are circulating in the blood. For example, when a certain amount of thyroid hormone is present in the bloodstream, the pituitary ceases production of thyroid-stimulating hormone until the level of thyroid hormone is reduced. Thus, the levels of circulating hormones are kept constantly in balance. This mechanism, known as negative feedback, is analogous to the system by which a thermostat is activated by room temperature to switch a furnace on or off.

Long-term administration from outside sources of adrenocortical, thyroid, or sex hormones causes virtual cessation of the corresponding stimulating hormone from the pituitary and, consequently, the eventual atrophy of the target gland. Conversely, if the output of a target gland is consistently subnormal, the constant production of the stimulating hormone from the pituitary causes an overgrowth of the gland, as in an iodine-deficiency goiter.

Hormone release is also regulated by the amount of certain substances in the bloodstream, the presence or utilization of which is under hormonal control. High levels of glucose in the blood stimulate the production and release of insulin, whereas low blood-sugar levels stimulate the adrenal glands to produce epinephrine and glucagon, maintaining an equilibrium in this aspect of carbohydrate metabolism. Similarly, a deficiency in blood calcium stimulates secretion of the parathyroid hormone, and a high blood-calcium level stimulates release of calcitonin from the thyroid.

Endocrine function is regulated also by the nervous system, as demonstrated by the adrenal responses to stress. The different endocrine organs are brought under nervous control in a variety of ways. The adrenal medulla and the posterior pituitary are richly innervated glands directly controlled by the nervous system. The adrenal cortex, thyroid, and gonads, however, although responding to various nervous stimuli, have no apparent nerve supply and continue to function when transplanted to other parts of the body. The anterior pituitary has a scanty nerve supply but cannot function if transplanted.

The way in which hormones exert their numerous metabolic and morphologic effects is not known. The effects on cell function, however, are thought to be caused either by action on cell membranes or on enzymes, by regulation of gene expression, or by control of the release of ions or other small molecules. Although apparently not consumed or changed in the metabolic process, hormones may be partly destroyed by chemical degradation. Hormonal end products are excreted rapidly and are found largely in the urine and also in feces and perspiration.

It's amazing to think that with all that is known about estrogen levels in females, and the clear effect the drop in estrogen has on the body of the average female, this area has been largely ignored by the majority of the medical profession.

The drop in estrogen levels after menopause does not only mean an end to a woman's reproductive years, but also a steep decline in many vital functions of the female body, an atrophy of several major body organs, a loss of interest and ability in sexual functioning and a much greater risk for the dreaded Alzheimer's Disease.

Interestingly, medical researchers know that while men see their testosterone levels drops after age 45 to 50, their estrogen levels actually begin to rise. One of the benefits in the increase of male estrogen levels appears to be less incidence of Alzheimer's Disease. Aging women are far more likely to develop Alzheimer's than men. They key is most likely estrogen.

When you combine the fact that loss of estrogen means not only a loss of a normal body for women, but also a possible loss of mind, looking more closely at estrogen replacement therapy becomes more urgent and more important than ever. And if combining estrogen with progesterone reduces estrogen's risk of cancer dramatically, it only makes sense that thousands more should be looking at estrogen replacement as a major option to all the agonies of a rapid decline of body and quality of life after menopause.

One of the most agonizing symptoms of menopause are the dreaded "hot flashes." This is an extremely unpleasant burst of intense heat in the body, followed by great discomfort and sweating. They last only a few minutes, but the aftereffects rob women of energy, and can cause them to lose an entire day that may have been otherwise enjoyable and productive. But sometimes, women can be tormented by multiple hot flashes, one coming right after another. In the latter case, we don't have to tell you that the effect on the woman who experiences it is distressing at best, and devastating at worst. Hot flashes can last two to five years after initial onset of menopause. Imagine five years of sudden attacks of debilitating body heat which leaves a person drained and distressed!

While this is going on, the estrogen starved female body has more to contend with. For starters, there is the thinning and drying of the vaginal walls. Sex becomes far less enjoyable, and can even lead to tearing and other damage of the vagina. Women also experience inexplicable mood swings, they feel constantly fatigued and drained of energy, their hair thins, their bones thin, making them weaker and more susceptible to broken hips or other bones, and even the skin wrinkles, adding years to the exterior look of a woman who might otherwise look years younger.

All of this can be turned around within a few weeks of replenishing the estrogen levels. Some of the beneficial effects can happen within days. Hot flashes stop completely. The vagina returns to its youthful feeling of being moisturized and resilient.

Sex drive returns to normal. Mood swings disappear. A feeling of youth and energy surges through he body. Even the hair becomes thicker, shiny and more luxurious, and the skin is smoothed of many wrinkles, and takes on a healthier, more youthful glow.

Even the most conservative doctors today agree that all of the above are the most common benefit of postmenopausal replacement of the female hormone in a woman's body. The problem is, however, that most of those same doctors will discontinue estrogen therapy after they feel a woman has gotten past her menopause years.

But all the research indicates there is no reason to stop estrogen therapy for years, if not decades, and perhaps for the rest of the lives of most women. One of the prime reasons is the prevention of major scourges for elderly women — bone thinning and Alzheimer's Disease.

Estrogen therapy can reduce the number of women who develop osteoporosis by a whopping fifty percent.

Osteoporosis is a bone condition characterized by a decrease in mass, resulting in bones that are more porous and more easily fractured than normal bones. Fractures of the wrist, spine, and hip are most common; however, all bones can be affected. White females are the most susceptible, but low calcium intake, inadequate physical activity, certain drugs (such as corticosteroids), and a family history of the disease are also risk factors.

The most common form of the disease, primary osteoporosis, includes postmenopausal, or estrogen-deficient, osteoporosis (Type I), which is observed in women whose ovaries have ceased to produce the hormone estrogen; age-related osteoporosis (Type II), which affects those over the age of 70; and idiopathic osteoporosis, a rare disorder of unknown cause that affects premenopausal women and men who are middle-aged or younger. Secondary osteoporosis may be caused by bone disuse as a result of paralysis or other conditions, including weightlessness in space; endocrine and nutritional disorders, including anorexia nervosa; specific disease processes; and certain drug therapies. Prevention and therapy of osteoporosis include estrogen or progestin therapy or both for postmenopausal women, intake of calcium and other nutrients, weight-bearing exercise, and new drugs such as calcitonin.

But estrogen may be the best "drug" of all. Taking estrogen can mean this disease never happens in the first place. Estrogen aids women in preserving their much-needed bone mass. And here's an extremely important point: All the best research indicates that osteoporosis can only be prevented if estrogen replacement is carried on for at least 10 years, not merely the three to five years most doctors allow for post menopausal women. Three to five years is probably not enough to save bone mass, and once bone mass is lost, replacing it is all but impossible.

Another piece of good advice is to get a bone density test done, whether you suspect you have a bone thinning problem or not. Women should have the knowledge they need about their own bodies so that

they can take action early to prevent problems far into the future, which, after they occur, may be too late to treat.

The best test is called the DEXA, which stands for Dual Energy X-Ray Absorptiometry. Because few doctors do this test as a matter of routine, you may have to ask for it. Your insurance may or may not pay for it. Still, having the knowledge this test provides will benefit you greatly down the line, and may prevent thousands of dollars in medical treatments in years to come and could even save your life.

Women over the age of 40 should also be involved in a regular exercise program. Light weightlifting is an excellent way to maintain and build bone and muscle mass, as well as reduce fat. Women who deplete calcium much faster than men need to have a daily high intake of calcium. Getting it through food is best, but a calcium supplement can't hurt and will only help. Women should also take vitamin D for healthy bones. All of these work with estrogen to ensure a strong, straight healthy female body full of energy and strength well into the far senior years.

Estrogen and the heart

Men get all the attention when it comes to heart disease. That's because the suffer from it earlier than women. Men are more often "cut down" in their prime by heart disease, which seems to make it an even greater tragedy than it already is. Because women more often suffer heart problems much later in life, the perception is that the problem is not as bad, since "she was already old anyway and past her best years."

But this is a lousy attitude toward women who die of heart disease when they could otherwise be enjoying many more years of youthful, healthy life despite advanced years.

The fact is, at least scientists believe it to be a fact, that estrogen prevents heart disease in aging women. Indeed, women who undergo hysterectomies and consequently lose their internal estrogen production levels, immediately begin to have three times as many heart attacks as women with normal estrogen levels. Does it not only seem like common sense to replace estrogen in women who have lost what they had and keep hundreds of thousands of them from dying?

Furthermore, estrogen can help women who have already have heart conditions. There are a number of studies which show that women who have been diagnosed with heart disease can increase their chances of not dying from it by 70 percent if they take estrogen. That's a much better chance than trying to go without. Loosely related to the issue of the heart is the cholesterol level of women. Estrogen lowers the level of bad cholesterol in women's blood, a major contributor to heart disease.

As we have mentioned elsewhere in this book, one of the prime contributors to the aging process is the breakdown of the body's DNA structure due to the presence of free radicals in the body. Scientists believe that certain food and vitamins, especially vitamin's A, E, C and beta-carotein, are very efficient free radical scrubbers in the body. But for the female body, perhaps a better free radical scrubber than all of the above is the hormone estrogen. It prevents free radical molecules from binding with DNA, thus halting one of the most common aspects of aging.

Estrogen also strengthens blood vessels, keeping them free from damage and blockages so that blood can flow without interruption to the heart and brain, helping keep them both healthy.

Speaking of a healthy brain, estrogen not only boosts the nutrient level of the brain and prevents a significant amount of Alzheimer's Disease in millions of women, it also helps with the flow of the brain's neurotransmitters, the very chemistry of thoughts themselves.

In the brain, electrical events propagate a signal within a neuron, the basic unit of the brain, or brain cell. Electricity and chemicals called neurostransmitters process the signals which leap from one neuron to another.

A neuron is a long cell that has a thick central area containing the nucleus; it also has one long process called an axon and one or more short, bushy processes called dendrites. Dendrites receive impulses from other neurons. (The exceptions are sensory neurons, such as those that transmit information about temperature or touch, in which the signal is generated by specialized receptors in the skin.) These impulses are propagated electrically along the cell membrane to the end of the axon. At the tip of the axon, the signal is chemically transmitted to an adjacent neuron or muscle cell.

A neuron is polarized, that is, it has a negative electrical charge inside the cell membrane. This is due to the free movement of positively charged potassium ions through the cell membrane and, at the same time, the retention of large, negatively charged molecules within the cell. Positively charged sodium ions are kept outside the cell by an active process. All cells have this charge difference, but when a stimulating current is applied to a nerve cell, a unique event occurs. First, potassium ions flow into the cell, reducing the negative charge (depolarization). At a certain point, the properties of the membrane change and the cell becomes permeable to sodium, which rapidly enters the cell and causes a net positive charge inside the neuron. This is called the action potential.

Once this potential is reached at one area in the neuron, it travels down the axon by ion exchange at specific points, called nodes of Ranvier. The size of the action potential is self-limiting because a high internal sodium concentration causes the pumping out first of potassium and then of sodium ions, restoring the negative charge inside the cell membrane; that is, the neuron is repolarized. The whole process takes less than one-thousandth of a second. After a very brief period, called the refractory period, the neuron can repeat this process.

When the electrical signal reaches the tip of an axon, it stimulates small presynaptic vesicles in the cell. These vesicles contain chemicals called neurotransmitters, which are released into the submicroscopic space between neurons. The neurotransmitters attach to specialized receptors on the surface of the adjacent neuron. This stimulus causes the adjacent cell to depolarize and propagate an action potential of its own. The duration of a stimulus from a neurotransmitter is limited by the breakdown of the chemicals in the synaptic cleft and the reuptake by the neuron that produced them. Formerly, each neuron was thought to make only one transmitter, but recent studies have shown that some cells make two or more.

In women, estrogen is the magic substance which keeps all this brain activity humming along normally. Among the most important of neurotransmitters is acetylcholine. Estrogen increases the amount of certain enzymes which are necessary for the production of acetylecholine in the brain.

Estrogen helps women retain strong memories. In addition to the hot flashes, mood swings and other miseries of menopause, many women find that their thinking becomes fuzzy, and that remembering certain words and names for some reason become more difficult. The answer for this memory problem lies in the hippocampus, the memory center of the brain. Estrogen binds to specific cells within the hippocampus allowing the growth of dendrites, which make up the net-like communication structure of the brain. Dendrite formation seems to decline as a regular aspect of aging, which is why older people seem to be more forgetful and are more prone to senile dementia.

It is interesting to note, however, that the reduction of dendrite formation in the brain is not so much a factor of physical aging as it is in the drop-off of normal brain use by elderly people.

After people retire, they tend to use their minds less. No longer having to perform the daily difficult tasks of getting a job done right, a retired person may spend more time with nonmental activities, such as watching TV, (the ultimate brain killer for a person of any age!) playing games that do not require a great deal of mental muscle, or just sitting around. As it turns out, it seems that the brain gets flabby with lack of use just as muscles do.

Studies have proven that old people who maintain mentally rigorous activities after retirement, such as reading, playing chess, solving problems, and more, see no decline in their ability to think clearly and have good memories. If you rest you rust. That's as true of the brain as it is of the rest of the physical body.

Thus, keeping the brain supplied with the nutrients it needs — oxygen, glucose, vitamins, enzymes which promote the production of essential neurotransmitters — and the all important hormones, in the case of women, estrogen is extremely important.

A healthy body without a healthy mind is not living in the true sense of youthfulness and vitality. One balances the other and completes the other.

What Is the Best Kind of Estrogen?

You may or may not know that not all estrogen drugs on the market are created equal. Some estrogens are derived from animals, most often horses. In fact, the most commonly prescribed estrogen is Premarin, which is extracted from the urine of pregnant horses. Yikes! And just think, you eat the stuff!

Many doctors feel that Premarin is not the best estrogen for many women. The main type of estrogen produced by the human female body is called estradiol, and Premarin contains only a small amount of this. There is a brand of estrogen manufactured which is primarily estradiol. Although it is a manufactured synthetic drug, and not an actual abstract of the human body, estradiol may be a closer match to what a woman needs. Estradiol may produce less of the harmful side effects of Premarin, including weight gain, headaches and possible more long-term effects, such as certain cancers. Still Premarin is not a bad drug; it's just the estradiol may be an even better choice for those who need to add estrogen to their biochemical system.

You can bet that medical science is working hard on finding even better forms of estrogen as the enormous and wide-ranging benefits of this are becoming ever more apparent.

A new class of drugs called SERM, which stands for selective estrogen receptor modulators, are under development as you read this, and some have already been tested on women with a variety of diseases. These drugs are sometimes called "smart estrogens" because they purportedly provide all the benefits of estrogen without the bad side effects. One such drug is called Tamoxifen, which is used to treat breast cancer. Tomixifan has drawbacks as well, however, which still do not make it a good choice for a replacement to more common estrogen drugs, such as Premarin. Another smart estrogen currently being tested is Raloxifene, which should receive FDA approval for use in the United States soon. But Raloxifene still may not be the final answer in the quest for the ultimate smart estrogen.

But the research effort will be well worth the time, money and resources being spent on what medical researchers will eventually develop.

Imagine an estrogen that provides all the benefits — restored youth, protection against Alzheimer's Disease, prevention of osteoporosis, maintenance of sex drive, muscle mass and strength — without any of the possible drawbacks to the long-term use of this powerful hormone and essential ingredient of human life.

When such a drug is developed, it could revolutionize the lives of women everywhere, allowing them to live youthful, healthy vigorous lives well into 100, 110, 120 or more years! The average death age of the American female, about 76, will then be considered mere middle age. We are closer than you think. Because of the promise of estrogen and other superhormones, the future is almost here.

NOTES

Chapter 5

Progesterone

One cannot talk about preserving or restoring the youth of females with estrogen without also telling the rest of the story. **The rest of the story concerns estrogen's best friend — pro gesterone.**

Mother Nature intended for estrogen to work hand-in-hand with progesterone. At their youthful peak, the biochemistry of a woman is in perfect balance, and the level of both estrogen and progesterone are at optimum levels and in balance with each other.

"I was taking estrogen for three years, and doing a lot better than I had before I started taking the drug, but I had other problems associated with estrogen that took the glow off the benefits I was receiving. Then my doctor prescribed progesterone to go along with my estrogen replacement therapy, and my life completely changed. Suddenly I felt like I was 35 years old again, even though I turn 75 next month! The balance of estrogen and progesterone in my body has made me stronger by making my bones stronger. I feel happier, and I almost never have a depressed or low mood anymore. I feel clear-headed, and I have the sex drive of a college girl — quite a thing to say for being three-quarters of a century old!"

— Bonnie H.
Newark, NJ

Almost an unknown, and relegated to the remote backwaters of endocrinological research, progesterone is a little studied substance which major pharmaceutical companies are not interested in. That's because progesterone is a natural substance manufactured within the human body and not a sexy new synthetic compound that can rake in shiploads of cash for the corporate greed heads of the world.

Progesterone is produced in large amounts by a woman's placenta during pregnancy, and if it didn't, the woman's baby would not come to term. As it's name implies, progesterone is heavily involved in the process of gestation. It is also produced in the adrenal glands and the corpus luteum.

Progesterone also helps regulate the menstrual cycle in women, and in fact, menstruation itself could not happen without this essential regulating hormone.

Low levels of progesterone have been linked to that dreaded plague which torments millions of women, PMS, or premenstrual syndrome. This condition has all the hallmarks of hormone imbalances — moodiness, headaches, bloating, cravings for sweet and fatty foods, nausea and a few others.

As with the other major hormones, progesterone levels decline in women as they age, often as early as age 30. The result is erratic menstrual cycles, more problems with PMS, depression and more. After menopause, progesterone production in the body practically ceases.

Since progesterone has such a close relationship with estrogen, it seems only common sense that when postmenopausal women are placed on estrogen therapy, they should also be given supplements of progesterone. After all, what is estrogen without progesterone? That's a good question. Part of the answer is that estrogen without progesterone is a major cancer causer! Progesterone balances the action of estrogen in a number of areas, perhaps most importantly in the area of uterine cancer. When women take only estrogen, the lining of the uterus thickens and grows. Without progesterone to induce a discharge of excess uterine tissue, much like a normal period, the result could be cancer of the uterus.

This further points out the fallacy of the "magic bullet" approach to medicine — simply trying to treat one thing, one organ, one imbalance, without looking at the whole system. A reductionist approach to medicine has long been the dominant strategy in treating the human body and in investigating new ways to cure diseases and bring people back to health. Reductionism refers to breaking things down into parts, and then examining these parts one at a time to greater understand the whole system. This is a highly effective and powerful method of exploration and learning. It's drawback,

however, is when reductionism becomes too dominant and scientists and doctors forget that human
beings are complex arrangements of interacting
chemicals of all kinds. When one goes out of balance, the rest are affected.

Thus, at first, doctors added progesterone simply
to counter the negative effects of estrogen, but they
soon discovered that replenishing formerly depleted
levels had a lot of other positive effects on the overall health of women.

Among those positive effects is a lowering of cholesterol levels and making weight gain and heart disease less likely in post menopausal women.

<u>Progesterone is definitely a bone builder.</u> Studies
show that women who supplement their body's with
progesterone stop losing bone mass and may even
regain lost bone mass.

In studies with animals progesterone clearly has
demonstrated that it cannot only prevent the loss of
bone mass, but can make bones grow bigger and
stronger, something which estrogen cannot do on its
own.

Better yet, the same effect has been observed in
humans. In one study which followed more than 100
women who had already undergone menopause, and
who were showing major to minor symptoms of
osteoporosis, three years of estrogen and progesterone therapy not only stopped the loss of bone
mass, but left all of the women with thicker stronger
bones. It should be noted that hormone replace-

ment therapy was not the only treatment applied to this group of women. They were also given calcium supplements, vitamins A, C, D and E, and they were forbidden to smoke or drink alcohol. They were also put on regular, guided exercise routines, including weight lifting, which has been proven to help build both muscle and bone mass.

It should be noted as well that while scientists believe the latter part of the treatment all helped, doing all these good things without also supplementing the body with hormones estrogen and progesterone may have not been enough to stop bone thinning and regrow new bone.

Another exciting area of possibility related to progesterone replacement therapy is the possibility that it may be a weapon against the very dreaded disease of multiple sclerosis and other diseases of the nerves.

Multiple Sclerosis is a disease of the central nervous system in which myelin, the white, fatty substance that sheathes nerve fibers, is gradually destroyed, and multiple lesions develop in the brain and spinal cord. The cause of the disease, which chiefly attacks individuals between the ages of 20 and 40, is unknown. Symptoms vary according to the sites of the lesions in the nervous system; the commonest symptoms are blurring of vision, loss of vision or double vision, tremor of the hands, weakness of the extremities, sensory changes such as numbness, tingling, or pain, slurring of speech, and loss of control over the urinary and anal sphincters.

The disease is intermittent in most cases; the initial symptoms are usually transient and may last only several hours or a few days. They generally disappear after the first attack, leaving the person symptom-free, often for many years, only to recur and disappear again, fully or partly. This waxing and waning of symptoms, which may vary from relapse to relapse, may occur repeatedly over many years, leaving few aftereffects at first but eventually producing permanent disabilities. Thus the person often becomes clumsy and progressively weaker. Occasionally, the disease is slowly progressive. It is rarely present as an acute or subacute condition running a progressive course of only weeks or months. Multiple sclerosis is in most cases eventually fatal; and no specific cure has been found. Physical and occupational therapy and several drugs may provide symptomatic improvement.

Progesterone is an extremely important element in allowing the central nervous system to operate normally and at top efficiency.. Progesterone is actually produced in special nerve cells called Schwan cells, found in the peripheral nerve system. When progesterone was added to the systems of MS patients, researchers observed that there was a significant increase in the myelin coating over the nerves.

In experiments with animals in which drugs were given to block the production of progesterone, a thinning and destruction of the myelin sheath was observed. It seems obvious, then, that progesterone plays a major role in maintaining healthy nerve fibers in the human body.

By the way, another important substance in promoting healthy myelin coatings for the nerves is vitamin B12.

Also known as cobalaminvitamin, B12 is necessary in minute amounts for the formation of nucleoproteins, proteins, and red blood cells, and for the functioning of the nervous system. Cobalamin deficiency is often due to the inability of the stomach to produce glycoprotein, which aids in the absorption of this vitamin. Pernicious anemia results, with its characteristic symptoms of ineffective production of red blood cells, faulty myelin synthesis, and loss of epithelium of the intestinal tract. Cobalamin is obtained only from animal sources, including liver, kidneys, meat, fish, eggs, and milk. That's why vegetarians would do well to take vitamin B12 supplements.

Thus, like a lot of other important vitamins, such as A, E, C and D, mixing progesterone with vitamin B12 brings about a variety of protective, regenerative and positive changes to the human body.

The largest tragedy about progesterone is lack of scientific study and interest being invested in this potential fountain of youth substance. As we said earlier, progesterone is not a big money maker for anyone.

Anyone can buy progesterone in any health food store, it comes in a variety of forms, from creams to tablets. It's safe and inexpensive, but the benefits it may produce for women and victims of MS and other neurophysiological disorders make it an even greater bargain, if not a downright miracle sub-stance. In the case of progesterone, we can say one of the best things in life is easy to obtain without great cost or any other kind of struggle.

Progesterone appears to be another golden key to the door that opens to a long life of health and youthful vigor.

NOTES

_____

_____

_____

_____

_____

_____

_____

_____

_____

_____

_____

Chapter 6

Thyroid Hormone

When a young person suffers from a hormone imbalance related to the thyroid, the symptoms are obvious and quickly remedied. But when an elderly person experiences many of the same symptoms — constant fatigue, poor thinking, clumsiness, minor aches and pains, hypersensitivity to cold — it is more often written off as just "old age."

It's true that thyroid hormone levels decline with age, and that most doctors feel this is natural and should not be changed unless a person is having great difficulty. But many people are being deprived of a higher quality of living and lifestyle because their doctors choose to let Mother Nature have its way and decline to put a patient's hormones back into youthful balance.

"I was 38 years old, but I felt like I was 98. That's no exaggeration. After a full 10 hours of sleep, I woke up in the morning feeling like an 18-wheel truck had run over me. All day I was listless, fatigued, clumsy, and my mind was cloudy. I would describe my life before thyroid hormone as one of pervasive and low-grade agony. I suffered from a million small agonies which, all added together, made my life a living hell. I was a classic picture of a man in failing health. My career as a high pressure journalist was all but over. The daily challenge of a newspaper reporter is tough enough on a healthy person, but for a person in my condition, it was next to impossible. Then my doctor discovered I was low on thyroid hormone. I was treated .. and WOW! I had my life back! I just can't describe to you the change I felt. I went from a pathetic slouch to a super-energized journalist who could outwork any 22-year-old cub reporter. What a godsend thyroid hormone has been for me. For me, it means life itself."

—Cory Marmota, 38,
Indianapolis, IN

Before we go on, it will be helpful to learn more about the thyroid gland and thyroid hormone and what is does for the human body

The thyroid gland is an endocrine gland found in almost all vertebrate animals and so called because it is located in front of and on each side of the thyroid cartilage of the larynx. It secretes a hormone that controls metabolism and growth.

The thyroid gland in human beings is a brownish-red organ having two lobes connected by an isthmus; it normally weighs about about 1 ounce and consists of cuboidal epithelial cells arranged to form small sacs known as vesicles or follicles. The vesicles are supported by connective tissue that forms a framework for the entire gland. In the normal thyroid gland, the vesicles are usually filled with a colloid substance containing the protein thyroglobulin in combination with the two thyroid hormones thyroxine, also called tetraiodothyronine **(T4),** and triiodothyronine **(T3).** These hormones are composed of the amino acid tyrosine, containing four and three iodine atoms, respectively.

The amount of thyroglobulin secreted by the thyroid is controlled by the thyroid-stimulating hormone **(TSH)** of the pituitary gland. Pituitary TSH, in turn, is regulated by a substance called thyroid-stimulating hormone releasing factor **(TRF),** which is secreted by the hypothalamus. Thyroglobulin is especially rich in iodine. Although the thyroid gland constitutes about 0.5 percent of the total human body weight, it holds about 25 percent of the total iodine in the body, which is obtained from food and water in the diet. Iodine usually circulates in the blood as an inorganic iodide and is concentrated in the thyroid to as much as 500 times the iodide level of the blood.

The primary hormone secreted by the thyroid gland is called thyroxine, also known as tetraiodothyronine, or **T4** for short. The function of this and the other thyroid hormone, triiodothyronine **(T3),** is to increase the cellular rate of carbohydrate metabolism and of protein synthesis and breakdown. The hormones are synthesized in the thyroid by combining iodine with the amino acid tyrosine and are secreted into the blood as a complex with the protein plasma globulin. Both synthesis and secretion are regulated by, and in turn regulate the formation of, a hormone secreted by the pituitary gland. Thyroxine was first isolated in 1919 by the American biochemist Edward Calvin Kendall and was synthesized in 1927 by the British bio-chemist Charles Harington. Synthetic thyroxine is now used in treating thyroid-deficiency conditions such as cretinism and goiter.

Closely associated with the thyroid gland is the parathyroid gland, which are any of a group of glan-dular cell aggregations located in the neck region close to the thyroid. In humans, four such clumps are usually present as distinct, yellowish-brown, encapsulated organs, each about six inches long. The combined weight of these glands is no more than 1/50 of an ounce. They are located beneath the thyroid gland; one or more of them are occasionally embedded in the thyroid tissue. Sometimes they may appear in association with the thymus, or any-where between the thyroid and thymus, or even else-where in the neck or upper anterior chest. Such glands, which may be present in addition to four nor-mally placed ones, are known as accessory parathy-roid tissue.

The parathyroid glands secrete a hormone known as Parathyroid hormone, which controls the concen-tration of calcium (calcium ion) and phosphorus (phosphate) in the blood. Calcium and phosphorus normally have a relationship to each other that the body keeps fairly constant. Parathyroid hormone acts to increase the excretion of phosphorus by the kidneys (which tends to lower blood phosphorus levels) and to increase the rate of resorption of cal-cium from bone (which tends to raise the level of blood calcium). Deficiency of Parathyroid hormone, which rarely occurs spontaneously and which is sometimes caused by accidental removal of the parathyroid glands during surgical excision of the thyroid, results in reduction of blood calcium, increase of blood phosphorus, and increased nervous excitability leading to rapid involuntary contractions of the muscles, a condition known as tetany. The accessory parathyroid tissue is occasionally sufficient to prevent severe deficiency symptoms when the essential four clumps are removed.

Unless accessory tissue is formed or hormone injections are given, Parathyroid hormone deficiency results in death. Overactivity of the parathyroid glands, occurring in cases of parathyroid tumors or hyperplasia of the normal glands, results in decreased blood phosphorus and increased blood calcium; the calcium in the bloodstream is withdrawn from the bones, which become soft as a result. Crystallization of excess calcium excreted in the urine in hyperparathyroidism may cause formation of kidney stones. The calcium may be carried to and deposited in the soft tissues of the body by the bloodstream; calcium deposition may also cause dysfunction of various organs, particularly the kidneys.

When Things Go Wrong with the Thyroid

Many different laboratory tests, including direct measurement of thyroxine and triiodothyronine, are used to test the activity of the thyroid gland. Thyroid scanning with radioiodine or technetium-99m is especially useful for detecting or ruling out cancer of the thyroid in persons who have a palpable nodule, or thyroid lump. In most cases thyroid cancers are slow-growing and not fatal. The thyroid gland appears to be quite sensitive to irradiation: during the 1970s an increased incidence of thyroid cancer was found among people who had been treated early in life with X rays for such conditions as acne, ringworm, and tonsillitis.

Excessive production of thyroid hormones, called hyperthyroidism or Graves' disease, results in elevated metabolism and activity. Sometimes this condition is associated with abnormalities of the eye, including bulging eyes. The usual treatment is to administer an antithyroid drug, such as propylthiouracil, or a dose of radioactive iodine, which is concentrated in the thyroid gland and destroys some of the tissue. Apparent hyperthyroidism can result from destruction of thyroid cells with release of large amounts of hormone. In one condition, called Hashimoto's thyroiditis, this destruction results from production of an antibody against thyroid tissue.

Deficiency of thyroid hormones, or hypothyroidism, is characterized by lethargy and lowering of metabolism. This condition can result from disorders of the pituitary or of the thyroid gland itself. Formerly a major cause of hypothyroidism in the Great Lakes and inland mountain areas of the U.S. was a deficiency of iodine in the diet, which caused a condition called goiter. Iodide is now added to table salt to prevent this. The condition called cretinism, more properly known as congenital hypothyroidism, is an inherited deficiency to thyroid function that occurs in about one in every 6000 births. In most instances, but not all, these infants grow up to be mentally retarded. Since early treatment can prevent retardation, Canadian researchers developed a test to detect the condition in newborns. Programs in Quebec and in the northeastern U.S. have been effective in limiting the effects of this abnormality.

Another thyroid problem is called myxedema. This is a swelling, deficiency disease caused by insufficient or lack of production of hormone by the thyroid gland. Patients with myxedema complain of fatigue, lethargy, sleepiness, poor tolerance to cold, mental sluggishness, a tendency to gain weight, and generalized aches and pains. Their faces often look puffy and waxy. Their skin is dry and coarse; their hair is coarse, dry, and brittle, and it tends to fall out easily. Often patients also lose the outer portion of their eyebrows. These and other symptoms are caused by a low metabolic rate resulting from a deficiency of the thyroid hormone that stimulates metabolism. Myxedema differs from cretinism in that it develops after birth and produces less severe cerebral inadequacy. The disease may occur in several members of a single family. Any condition that decreases the elaboration of thyroid gland hormone may bring on myxedema. The disease is treated by the administration of thyroxine, other thyroid extracts, or a synthetic preparation such as levothyroxine.

No discussion of thyroid problems would be complete without mention of one of the most well-known and agonizing thyroid gland disorders — goiters. **There are two kinds of goiters, simple goiters and toxic goiters.**

Simple Goiter

This is an enlargement of the entire gland, or of one of its two lobes, caused by a deficiency of iodine in the diet. The disease is especially apt to appear in adolescence. Simple goiter occurs in inland areas of all continents. It was common in what was at one time referred to as the goiter belt of the U.S., which includes the Great Lakes region and inland mountain areas. The administration of iodine, or of the iodine-containing hormone thyroxine, effectively prevents the disease. Prevention requires taking small doses of iodine for long periods. Ingestion of iodine during pregnancy prevents development of the disease in the infant as well as in the mother. Public health measures, including the addition of iodine to water supplies and to table salt, have helped to reduce the incidence of simple goiter in certain areas. Iodine is most effective when administered to children who have the disease. Thyroidectomy, or surgical removal of the gland, may be necessary in cases in which the gland has become greatly enlarged.

Toxic Goiter

This disease, also called exophthalmic goiter, hyperthyroidism, thyrotoxicosis, or Graves' disease, for the 19th Century Irish physician Robert James Graves, is caused by an excess of thyroxine secretion. The cause of the excessive secretion is obscure. In some cases it may result from excessive stimulation by the pituitary gland. The symptoms of toxic goiter may include a rapid heartbeat, tremor, increased sweating, increased appetite, weight loss, weakness, and fatigue. Some patients have eye problems, such as staring or protrusion. Thiouracil and iodine are sometimes used in the treatment of toxic goiter, as is irradiation of the gland by radioactive iodine.

How to Tell if You Are Hormone Deficient

You don't have to have a goiter the size of a football on your neck to know that you have a problem with your thyroid.

Doctors diagnose thyroid hormone deficiency with a blood test. If you have a high TSH level, it may mean that your pituitary gland is trying to stimulate your thyroid gland to get it to produce more hormone. Doctors will also look at T3 and T4.

Sometimes, however, all the numbers can look normal, yet the person still displays all the symptoms of a thyroid disorder. In that case, few doctors will recommend medication to replace low thyroid hormone levels. But you can do some additional tests on your own to get to the bottom of things. For one, you can take your basal temperature. You do this by placing a thermometer under your arm immediately after you wake up. If your temp is below 97.4 Fahrenheit, it may be a sign that your thyroid hormone levels are out of balance.

Many people are also depressed and forgetful, for no apparent reason. Some people who are depressed fail to respond to popular antidepression drugs such as Prozac and trycyclics. At the same time, these people may have everything going well in their daily lives, yet they feel inexplicably bad about things. In these cases, low thyroid levels may be the cause. In fact, low thyroid levels may be a major contributors to America's No. 1 mental health problem — depression. Supplementing the body chemistry with thyroid hormone can bring back a clear mind, chase away the blues, and make a person "feel like himself."

If having a cloudy mind and being depressed is not enough, low thyroid hormone levels leave you open to more diseases because it slows down your immune system. Thyroid hormone stimulates the formation of lymphocytes, cells which attack invading germs in the body. People become more susceptible to diseases as they get old, and again, most doctors simply consider this to be a "natural" aspect of getting old. But perhaps this doesn't have to be. By replenishing dwindling thyroid hormone levels and the other superhormones, an elderly person can have the same powerful immune system that a young person has naturally.

A final note about thyroid hormone replacement therapy: It is probably better to take natural hormone as opposed to synthetic hormones. There are two kinds of synthetic, or man-made hormones generally prescribed by doctors. One is called Synthoid, which contains T4 only. Another is called Cytomel and it contains T3. But there is an animal-based product called desiccated thyroid hormone which contains both T3 and T4. Many doctors believe this form of thyroid hormone is superior to the two synthetic products we mentioned because it is more complete and is produced biologically, rather than in a laboratory.

If you are over the age of 35, we urge you to see your doctor and discuss your thyroid levels with him or her. Doing so may be the key to a rejuvenated life of high energy, freedom from disease, clear thinking, and a general feeling of well-being and a forward looking attitude toward each day that greets you in the morning.

Growth Hormone

Now let's turn our attention to something called growth hormone, a potentially miraculous substance which has been the subject of intense medical research and a source of sky-high hopes among a large body of elderly people.

Some say growth hormone is the veritable Fountain of Youth itself, while others believe it is definitely being overbilled.

It's important to know, since those who want to take growth hormone will have to shell out some $10,000 a year. Yes, it's extremely expensive, and it might be worth it if it actually performed everything it promises to do for the human body — namely, prevent it from getting old.

Growth hormone is a substance necessary for human growth. It is produced naturally in the human body by the anterior lobe of the pituitary gland. The hormone affects uptake of amino acids and metabolism of fats. It also stimulates secretion by the liver of the hormone somatomedin, which carries out bone formation. Secretion of growth hormone is increased by exercise, stress, and lowered glucose intake and by insulin and the estrogens. Release of growth hormone is inhibited by a protein called somatostatin, which is produced by the hypothalamus, a brain structure that probably also produces a factor that stimulates the release of growth hormone.

There are several well-known diseases associated with abnormal growth hormone production levels in some people, the most common being gigantism and dwarfism.

Gigantism is caused by an excess of the hormone during childhood. In humans, when gigantism begins in childhood, before normal ossification has been completed, it is usually caused by overactivity of the anterior pituitary gland in production of the growth hormone. Hereditary defects that prevent normal ossification at the time of puberty, and thus permit continued growth, may also cause a type of gigantism. Because the growth hormone depresses the secretory powers of the gonads, gigantism is often accompanied by weakened sexual function and is then called eunuchoid gigantism. Gigantism may occur, however, without disturbance in sex function. Individuals affected by either type of gigantism are muscularly weak. Acromegaly, a related condition caused by excessive production of the pituitary growth hormone, occurs in the third decade of life. It usually results in excessive growth of the hands, feet, and chin.

Overproduction syndromes appear to respond to administration of somatostatin, and dwarfism to administration of growth hormone. Scientists recently developed a process for making human growth hormone by genetic engineering, and several drugs are now available to treat children with short stature resulting from a deficiency of growth hormone.

Dwarfism is caused by underproduction of the hormone in childhood. The result is an undersized body, sometimes called dwarfism. Some dwarfs have been less than 64 cm (24 in) tall when fully grown. The term midget is usually applied to physically well-proportioned dwarfs. The term pygmy is applied to people whose shortness of stature is a racial trait and not the result of pathological conditions.

Cretinism, a result of a disease of the thyroid gland, is the cause of most dwarfism in Europe, Canada, and the United States. Other causes of dwarfism are Down's syndrome, a congenital condition with symptoms similar to those of cretinism; achondroplasia, a disease characterized by short extremities resulting from absorption of cartilaginous tissue during the fetal stage; spinal tuberculosis; and deficiency of the secretions of the pituitary gland or of the ovary.

Treatment of cretinism with thyroxine or thyroid extract early in infancy results in normal growth and development. Pituitary dwarfism is successfully treated by administering human growth hormone.

Another disease called acromegaly is a chronic disease marked by overgrowth of the hands, feet, and lower part of the face, resulting from excessive production of somatotropin, the growth-stimulating hormone. In many cases, over secretion of the hormone can be traced to a tumor of the pituitary gland. Acromegaly is accompanied by progressive weakness and sometimes by diabetes mellitus; on occasion it occurs during lactation. The disease usually appears in adulthood and frequently affects more than one member of a family. Treatment consists of microsurgical removal of hyperfunctioning tissue, pituitary irradiation, and drugs that suppress growth hormone. A similar disorder, gigantism, occurs in children, producing overgrowth of the long bones of the body. A deficiency in growth hormone production results in dwarfism, a condition marked by abnormally short bone development.

Still another disease associated with growth hormone is cretinism, a deficiency disease caused by congenital absence of thyroxine, a hormone secreted by the thyroid gland, and characterized by defective mental and physical development. Cretins have dwarfed bodies, with curvature of the spine and pendulous abdomen. Their limbs are distorted, their features are coarse, and their hair is harsh and scanty. Mental development is retarded throughout life. An adult cretin may reach the intelligence of only a four-year-old child. Research has revealed that when an animal or human infant is born with a deficiency of thyroxine, the neurons (nerve cells) in the brain do not develop the multiple branches that normally form the brain's complex network. Treatment of adult cretins with thyroxine or thyroid extract results in some improvement; early treatment in infancy results in cure of the disease and normal development of the individual, provided the treatment is continued throughout life. Treatment is sometimes begun prenatally, for instance, when a mother suffers from severe goiter, a disease of the thyroid.

Endemic cretinism is found associated with goiter throughout the world, especially in certain valleys of the Alps and Pyrenees mountains, and in Syria, India, and China. Families moving into such areas tend to develop goiter in the first generation and cretinism in the second and succeeding generations. Public health measures, including the addition of iodine to public water supplies, have proved beneficial in reducing the incidence of goiter and cretinism in certain areas. Iodine is an essential building block of thyroxine.

But for people with normal growth hormone levels and none of the diseases described above, is there any reason to supplement your body chemistry with more growth hormone?

The answer is probably no. First of all, as we have said, growth hormone is extremely expensive. But perhaps more importantly, it can produce some unwanted side effects.

Third, and perhaps most importantly, you should have little need to take growth hormone artificially if you are already supplementing your personal body chemistry with the other super hormones we have already discussed at length throughout this book.

Fourth, you can stimulate the natural production of growth hormone in your body by exercising vigorously and on a regular basis. As we will discuss in more detail later in this book, exercise in and of itself has almost miraculous effects on the aging process. One of the major reason regular exercise can slow down the aging process is the fact that it stimulates the production of growth hormone.

The level of growth hormone production in our bodies declines by about 15 percent for every 10 years we age. By age 60, the human body produces only tiny amounts of the stuff. Stress and diseases can also block the production of this necessary hormone. This is part of the reason people over the age of 60 experience all the common effects of aging — loss of muscle mass, bone thinning, loss of hair, wrinkled skin, loss of energy and strength, and more.

The people who will most benefit from growth hormone supplements are probably those who are already sick with the common diseases of old age. As we have already stated, starting on a regular regimen of the other superhormones may prevent the need for growth hormone supplement in the first place, but for those older people who did not have the benefit of this knowledge a few years ago, growth hormone may be able to make up for some of the lost ground they have already suffered.

Growth hormone may be one of the only known substances that can cause muscles to actually regrow in the body. Growth hormone not only helps increase muscle mass in healthy people who exercise, but may aid in bringing back muscle to people who are generally too weak to exercise, or who need a boost to make their exercise regimen more effective. So while growth hormone is not for everyone, those who have specific problems with loss of muscle mass may benefit greatly from this hormone.

In addition to helping out with muscles, growth hormone can be a key to healthy kidneys. As we age, the kidneys tend to function less efficiently. People become more prone to kidney failure with old age. But growth hormone can help by decreasing the amount of nitrogenous wastes passing through the kidneys, making them more efficient and letting them carry less of a burden. Growth hormone may reduce the need for dialysis which many people must undergo one to three times a week. For those of you who may not know, kidney dialysis is also known as hemodialysis and is a medical treatment used to remove waste materials from the blood of patients lacking renal function. Blood from an artery is pumped through a dialyzer, or artificial kidney, where it flows past a semipermeable membrane. Dialysis fluid passing on the other side of the membrane removes unwanted elements in the blood by diffusion. The blood is then returned to the body through a vein.

Eliminating the need or just the frequency of dialysis in and of itself would be a major benefit.

Another very particular situation in which growth hormone may play an important role is in fighting heart disease. Remember that growth hormone has the effecting of building and improving muscle. Well, the heart is basically one big muscle, perhaps the most important muscle in the human body. The older we get, the thicker the heart tends to become, losing the efficiency with which it pumps blood, supplying the body with oxygen, glucose and other nutrients of the blood. The same condition can develop in young people as the result of disease.

This condition is called cardiomyopathy and is usually treated with digitalis, the drug made from the foxglove plant. In some cases, however, much of the heart can become so damaged from cardiomyopathy, that the only option is a heart transplant. Medical researchers know that young people who are susceptible to cardiomyopthy are low in natural levels of growth hormone. Thus, in these cases, growth hormone may do more to strengthen the heart than does digitalis, and may make the heart strong enough so that it goes back to being a good old "normal" heart.

Many studies have already been done which strongly indicate that growth hormone is indeed an effective treatment for cardiomyopthy. Heart patients given growth hormone were able to cut down on their intake of digitalis while seeing dramatic improvement in the function of their hearts at the same time.

In addition to making the heart stronger, growth hormone has been shown to lower the level of bad cholesterol in the human body. Too much cholesterol is one of the major causes of heart disease in America today. People who take growth hormone not only see a reduction in the cholesterol levels, but they also lose weight, lose body fat and gain positive muscle mass. Furthermore, growth hormone seems to have the effect of redistributing fat in the body in such a way that it takes it away from where it is most unwanted, and puts it where it is more needed. The result is a much more attractive physical appearance.

The negative side effects of growth hormone are carpal tunnel syndrome, diabetes and severe fluid retention. Most medical researchers agree that administering growth hormone should be limited to those people with very specific problems which the hormone can go directly to work on. Also, people in their 40s, 50s, 60s or older should have little reason to take this hormone, especially when they have the options of DHEA, estrogen, testosterone, pregnenolone, progesterone, thyroid hormone and others on hand to take care of just about all the problems of aging.

One of the future keys to gaining all the benefits of growth hormone without any of its side effects is a new drug being developed by researchers which will stimulate the body's natural production of its own growth hormone, eliminating the need for artificial growth hormone supplements. This new drug is one of a class of substances that are being called growth-hormone-releasing agents.

When will they be available? Probably not until the year 2005, or so, although actual experiments on human beings are taking place as this book is being written. Most drugs take 10 to 15 years to reach the general market, although some see a rather rapid journey from the lab to the general market. Prozac, for example, was available to the general public through a doctor's prescription in less than 10 years after its first development. If we're lucky, growth-hormone-releasing agents will follow the same rapid road as did other so called "miracle" drugs like Prozac.

Chapter 7

Miracle Melatonin

Perhaps no other over-the-counter health supplement has generated as much public and
press excitement as melatonin has in the past
five years. Hardly a newspaper, radio station or TV
news team has not done a dozen major stories or
more on this substance in the past two years.

Melatonin is flying off the shelves of health food
stores as fast as manufacturers can produce the
stuff. New formulations and dosage levels are being
introduced to the market on a daily basis, and millions of people are swearing that melatonin is everything it is being hyped to be.

So what is this miracle substance, and what can it really do for human beings?

Does it extend life, as many claim it does? Does it
stop the aging process, or at least slow it down? Is it
the best cure for insomnia on the market? Does
melatonin bring your body back into some kind of

heavenly balance that will make all your aches and pains go away, cure your diseases, and make you feel like a millions dollars every single day of the week?

Lots of claims, lotst of questions, but the answers to many of those questions seem contradictory or so filled with hype and wild claims that it's difficult to know what to believe.

But we think it is safe to say that melatonin does these things:

- Helps you live longer
- Makes you feel and look younger longer
- Improves your sex life
- Boosts your immune system
- Scrubs harmful free radicals from your body
- Fights the physical effects of stress
- Can prevent cancer
- Stops heart disease
- Is a natural cure for insomnia
- Effective remedy for jet lag

Those are some tall claims for a a daily dose of a few milligrams of hormones, but increasing evidence suggests they all may be true. To understand why melatonin may be the true miracle many promise it to be, it will be helpful to go straight to the source of where melatonin is made — in the human brain. More specifically, melatonin is manufactured in a part of the brain called the pineal gland, what ancient mystics used to call the "Third Eye."

The pineal gland, sometimes called the pineal body, is a small, cone-shaped projection from the top of the midbrain of most vertebrates, arising embry-ologically as an outgrowth of the brain. Interestingly, the pineal gland is absent in crocodiles and in mammals of the order Edentata (anteaters, sloths, armadillos) and consists of only a few cells in whales and elephants. In humans the structure develops until the seventh year, when it is slightly larger than a pea; thereafter, throughout life, small mineral particles, particularly calcium, may be deposited in the pineal body. The mineral deposits can sometimes be seen in skull X-ray photographs.

Named after a French psychologist, Philippe Pinel, who first described the gland in the human brain in the early 1800s, it is only slowly beginning to be understood in its functions. It has both neural and endocrine properties, and in simple vertebrates such as the lamprey the organ is mounted on a stalk close to an opening in the skull and functions as a photoreceptive organ. Photoreceptive structures linked with the pineal body are still observed in higher vertebrates such as reptiles and even some species of birds. In mammals the pineal body is not light-sensitive, but a neural connection remains between the eyes and the gland. Thus the functions of the pineal body in an animal are linked with surrounding light levels.

It was 1958 when researchers discovered a substance called melatonin was actually manufactured by the pineal gland. This led to a further understanding of the pineal gland. Animal studies show that the gland synthesizes and secretes melatonin almost entirely at night, and that it ceases this function during the day. Melatonin, in turn, affects the functions of other endocrine organs such as the thyroid, adrenals, and gonads. Further experiments demonstrate that changes in the level of melatonin in the bodies of seasonally breeding animals affect their reproductive cycle, and that decreases in melatonin brought about by artificial lighting can prolong breeding activity. The role of the pineal body in the control of these biorhythms is only beginning to be elaborated, but the suggestion remains that even nonseasonal breeders such as human beings are affected by its daily functions. The onset of puberty may, in fact, be triggered by changes in melatonin level.

An extremely important aspect of the pineal gland and melatonin is setting the biological clocks of not only humans, but most animals. To help you understand how essential and vital melatonin is to our daily lives, let's look closer at biological clocks.

Biological clocks are physiological systems that enable organisms, including you, to live in harmony with the rhythms of nature, such as the cycles of day and night and of the seasons. Such biological clocks exist for almost every kind of periodicity throughout the plant and animal world, but most of what is known about them comes from the study of circadian, or daily, rhythms. Circadian rhythms cue typical daily behavior patterns even in the absence of external cues such as sunrise, demonstrating that such patterns depend entirely on internal timers for their periodicity.

No clock is perfect, however. When organisms are deprived of the cues the world normally provides, they display a characteristic "free-running" period of not quite 24 hours. As a result, free-running animals or human being drift slowly out of phase with the natural flow of things.

In experiments in which people are isolated for long periods of time, they continue to eat and sleep on regular but increasingly out-of-phase schedules. Such drift does not take place under normal circumstances, because external cues reset the clocks each day. Light is usually the most important cue, but many organisms can make use of rhythmic variations in temperature or other sensory inputs to readjust their internal timers. When a clock's error becomes large, however, complete resetting sometimes requires days. This phenomenon is well known to long-distance air travelers as jet lag.

The physiological circuitry underlying the use of external cues is quite simple; for example, a single flash of light can act as a trigger, signifying dawn. Research in the 1980s has suggested that such simple light-triggering extends even to the behavior of human beings. Research also suggests that, at least in some organisms, a single gene may underlie the mechanism of biological clocks. In the fruit fly, for example, a gene known as per (short for period) is required by the insect to maintain its biological rhythms. This gene has been found to code for a chemical called a proteoglycan, a long-chain molecule containing sugar units attached to a protein. Proteoglycans are also found in mammals.

Interestingly, biological clocks can exist in every cell and even in different parts of a cell. Hence, an isolated piece of tissue — for example, the eye of a sea slug — will maintain its own daily rhythm but will quickly adopt that of the whole organism when restored to it. In the brains of most animals a master clock appears to exist that communicates its timing signals chemically to the rest of the organism. For example, a brain removed from a moth pupa and exposed to an artificial sunrise of one time zone, then implanted into the abdomen of a headless pupa on a different time zone schedule, will cause the second pupa to emerge at the time of day appropriate to the disconnected brain floating in its abdomen.

The clock in the brain triggers the release of a hormone that switches on all the complex behavior involved in pupal emergence. In hamsters, experiments have shown a master biological clock to be located in the hypothalamus. The brain-cell groups are called suprachiasmatic nuclei.

Melatonin is also known to be involved in long-term biological rhythms. Besides being of scientific interest, a fuller understanding of biological clocks could be important in many ways. One promising theory of aging, for example, is based on an observation that, in old age, the many separate, subordinate clocks in the body seem somehow to become less tightly coupled to the master clock in the brain. This lack of synchronization may contribute to many of the problems associated with aging.

So we can see that melatonin is at the very base of the ryhthm of life itself, and is probably the "Master Key" to the aging process itself.

So melatonin has come under increasing investigation as an anti-aging substance, but it is also being looked at as a treatment for a number of other conditions having to do with biological clocks, including, jet lag, seasonal affective disorder (SAD), depression, and cancer. Furthermore, pineal polypeptide extract (which contains a broad spectrum of other protein-based pineal hormones) has been shown to inhibit the development of atherosclerosis, reduce blood triglyceride levels, improve cellular immunity, and increase lifespan in animals.

In the human body, melatonin levels peak at about 2 a.m. in normal, healthy young people, and at about 3 a.m. in elderly people. Melatonin production, like most other hormones, declines with age. By the time a person reaches age 65, they produce about 50 percent less than a youthful person age 22-35.

Also, and for young and old alike, melatonin levels are low during the day. At sunset, the end of light triggers neural signals which stimulate the pineal gland to begin releasing melatonin. This rise continues for hours, eventually peaking around 2 a.m. (3 a.m. for the elderly) after which it steadily declines to minimal levels by morning. The delay in timing and decrease in intensity of the melatonin pulse is a manifestation of the aging process.

Melatonin regulates many neuroendocrine functions. When the timing or intensity of the melatonin peak is disrupted (as in aging, stress, jet lag, or artificial jet lag syndromes), many physiological and mental functions are adversely affected. The ability to think clearly, remember key facts, and make sound decisions can be profoundly hampered by these upsets in the biological clock. All of these symptoms are associated with old age, and for old people, have been called "normal." But why should all these life-robbing problems be considered normal in any human being of any age who wants to live a full and happy life? Why not instead bring the melatonin levels back to their youthful levels, and let the rest of the hormones and regulators which depend on melatonin follow suit. Why not indeed. Before we discuss this more, let's look at a couple more specific problems which can be addressed effectively with melatonin.

Jet Lag

Jet lag happens when you mess with the biological clock. Confuse the biological clock, and you throw everything in your body out of whack. The result is that you feel like a truck has run over you. You are tired, mentally sluggish, have headaches, irritability, constipation, insomnia and you just feel completely run down. (Again, all classic symptoms many associate with old age). The modern era of travel in super fast jet airplanes has produced one of the most baffling dilemmas for the human hormone system ever encountered.

Jet lag is generally worse when flying in an easterly direction, and it may take as long as one day for each time zone crossed in order to fully recover. Not surprisingly, older people, who have less melatonin, have an even tougher time adjusting to these changes than younger people.

Jet travel is not the only way to throw off the biological clock. It can also be done by working night shifts, working rotating shifts (like physician-interns, management trainees for 24-hour businesses, and soldiers under battle-alert conditions), or by staying up all night. Whatever its causes, jet lag and artificial jet lag syndromes are seriously debilitating to cognitive function.

The answer for travelers is to take melatonin the evening of the new time zone you have traveled to. This rapidly resets the biological clock and will almost totally alleviate (or prevent) the symptoms of jet lag. The ability of melatonin to alleviate jet lag was demonstrated in a study of 17 subjects flying from San Francisco to London (eight time zones away). Eight subjects took 5 mg of melatonin, while nine subjects took a placebo. Those who took melatonin had almost no symptoms of jet lag.

Six out of nine placebo subjects scored above 50 on the jet lag scale, and all of the melatonin subjects scored below 17.

Most people sleep well with melatonin, and wake up the next day refreshed with no symptoms of jet lag (although they may still have some fatigue from the wear and tear of traveling).

Many melatonin fans without any noticeable symptoms of circadian disturbance are now using melatonin to enhance their circadian rhythms. They report that it helps them get to sleep and helps them sleep more soundly. It also makes them more alert the next day and even lessens mid-afternoon tiredness (and naps).

In all cases, melatonin should be taken at night (preferably before midnight) before going to bed. That's when your pineal gland naturally releases melatonin. Taking melatonin at night (or before your normal bedtime if you are a shift worker) helps restore and maintain normal circadian metabolic rhythms.

Melatonin and Mental Performance

At first, many researchers believed that melatonin disrupted the ability to think clearly — until they discovered that they were giving test subject doses of melatonin right before they were given tests! That's just like giving someone a sleeping pill and then expecting them to score 100 on a driving test. Remember, melatonin is produced in the human body at nighttime, when the body is ready for sleep. The brain likes melatonin during night hours and sleep time, but during the day when it's time to be clear and thinking, it does not want melatonin.

But the researchers wised up and tried giving subjects melatonin at night, and then testing them the following day after a good night's sleep. The results were that in just about all cases, mental ability was greatly improved.

This shows that with circadian enhancers like melatonin, the timing is critical. When taken in opposition to the body's natural circadian rhythm, they cause cognitive deficit just like jet lag does. But when taken in synchronization with the body's natural circadian rhythms, they enhance mental performance. By giving melatonin in the daytime, before the cognitive tests, the researchers were causing the test subjects to suffer from artificial jet lag and then measuring the resulting cognitive impairment. Disruption of circadian rhythms produces amnesia by interfering with the circadian organization of memory processes.

Melatonin, by correcting circadian rhythms should, theoretically, improve mental performance. We could only find one study in which melatonin was given to rats at night. This study confirmed that next-day measures of learning ability improved. We believe that melatonin, when taken before sleep, will decrease sleep disturbances of any kind, and will, therefore, improve mental function during the following day.

Melatonin for Depression

Two particularly notable features of depression and SAD are diminished nighttime release of melatonin and abnormal sensitivity to melatonin suppression by light. This has led researchers and clinicians to try melatonin as an experimental treatment for depression, with gratifying results.

Melatonin Extends Lifespan

Melatonin has also been shown to improve immunity and extend lifespan in rodents. In 1988, medical researchers gave melatonin to middle-aged mice each evening. The treated mice became healthier (better posture, increased activity levels, and thicker, more lustrous fur) and lived an average of 20% longer than control mice.

Melatonin secretion naturally drops off with age. This decrease is so reliable that blood melatonin levels have been proposed as a measurement of biological age. This age-related reduction in melatonin levels may partially account for the reason many older people have difficulty sleeping at night, and for why they are so fatigued during the day. We believe they may be suffering from age-induced "jet lag." Restoration of normal sleep-wake cycles in many elderly patients with supplemental melatonin before bedtime has dramatically improved their quality of life.

Melatonin: Anti-Stress Hormone

One of the primary ways the body ages and becomes less able to fend off disease is through stress. Just what kind of stress are we talking about, and what does it do to the human body and it's chemistry?

A pioneer in the study of stress was the Canadian physician Hans Selye, who died in 1982. Selye identified three stages in the stress response. In the first stage, alarm, the body recognizes the stress and prepares for action, either to fight or escape. Endocrine glands release hormones that increase heartbeat and respiration, elevate blood sugar, increase perspiration, dilate the pupils, and slow the digestion. In the second stage, resistance, the body repairs any damage caused by the alarm reaction. If the stress continues, however, the body remains alert and cannot repair the damage. As resistance continues, the third stage, exhaustion, sets in, and a stress-related disorder might result. Prolonged exposure to stress depletes the body's energy supplies and can even lead to death.

Stress problems commonly involve the autonomic nervous system, which controls the body's internal organs. Some kinds of headache and back and facial pain, asthma, stomach ulcers, high blood pressure, and premenstrual stress, or PMS, are examples of stress-related disorders.

Physicians have long recognized that people are more susceptible to diseases of all kinds when they are subjected to great stress. Negative events such as the death of a loved one seem to cause enough distress to lower the body's resistance to disease. Positive circumstances, however, such as a new job or a new baby in the house, can also upset a person's normal ability to fend off disease. Social scientists have devised a list of life events and rated the relative stressfulness of each. Thus, the death of a spouse rates a 100 on the scale, whereas trouble with one's employer rates 23; being fired, 47; going to jail, 63; a change in sleeping habits, 16; getting divorced, 73; and so on.

Although stress can exert some influence on any disease, such as a cold or tuberculosis and perhaps even cancer, it affects some disorders directly. Scientists attribute at least part of this effect to evolutionary history, reasoning that at one time people had to live with constant physical threats from wild animals and the elements, as well as from one another, and that the body developed in a way that helped it cope with these physical stresses. The heart beats faster, blood pressure rises, and other body systems prepare to meet the threat. When a person does something active to cope with a threat, these systems return to normal.

Running away or fighting — the famous flight or fight reaction — are both successful ways of coping with many physical threats. Problems arise, however, when the body is prepared, as described, to cope with danger but cannot do so. Being caught in a traffic jam, for example, can cause the body to prepare for a flight or fight response, but when no action can be taken, the body's systems remain overly active. Similar repeated experiences of this frustrating nature can lead to conditions such as high blood pressure.

Many other determinants also may lead to stress-related disorders. Among those under investigation is a certain type of behavior that scientists call "type-A," a term originally applied to people who are prone to coronary artery disease.

The type-A coping style, characterized by competitive, hard-driving intensity, is common in American society, and mounting evidence indicates that type-A behavior is associated with an increased incidence of several stress-related disorders.

High blood pressure, or hypertension, is one of the most common disorders made worse by stress. It afflicts an estimated 15 to 20 out of every 100 Americans. Although it has no noticeable symptoms, hypertension can damage the kidneys and can lead to stroke.

Other stress-related disorders that are even more common are gastrointestinal problems. More serious are peptic ulcers and anorexia nervosa. Ulcers are caused by an excess of gastric juices or unusual sensitivity in an area of the stomach lining, causing nausea and pain.

Anorexia nervosa, a disorder most common among adolescent girls, is characterized by a refusal to eat to the extreme that death may result. Other stress-related gastrointestinal disorders include inflammatory diseases of the colon and bowel, such as ulcerative colitis and regional enteritis.

Respiratory disorders also can be affected by stress. Most common of these is asthma, which may be caused by emotional upsets. Asthma attacks are characterized by wheezing, panting, and a feeling of being suffocated. In addition, emotional stress can cause or aggravate many skin disorders, from those that produce itching, tickling, and pain to those that cause rashes and pimples.

Major traumatic events such as accidents, catastrophes, or battle experiences may bring on a condition now called post-traumatic stress disorder (PTSD). Once known under war conditions as shell shock or battle fatigue, PTSD gained its current name after it appeared in many veterans returning from Vietnam as they tried to readjust to civilian life. Its symptoms, which may take months to appear after an initial state of numbness is observed, include nervous irritability, difficulty in relating to surroundings, and depression.

Melatonin to the Rescue

Now imagine a simple substance that could undo all of the above. All you have to do is swallow one every night before you go to bed, and when you wake up in the morning the slate is wiped clean — at least as far as your physical body is concerned.

Experiments were started with mice, which have remarkably similar brain structures to humans. In mice, taking melatonin at night showed that it could counteract the immune-suppressing effects of acute anxiety stress in mice. Measures used to confirm the positive effects on mice were measures of their thymus weight, antibody production, and ability to fight off a lethal viral infection.

In humans, melatonin appears to work with certain chemicals produced by the body's immune system, specifically, endorphins. These are peptides that act on the peripheral and central nervous systems to reduce sensitivity to pain. Peptides are one of a group of organic chemicals found in nearly all living tissues and having a wide range of biological functions.

The chemicals are relatively low-weight polymers of amino acids, as contrasted with the high-weight proteins. The acids are linked together by so-called peptide bonds between their carboxyl (COOH) and alpha amino (NH2) groups. Those peptides containing fewer than 10 amino acids are called oligopeptides; those containing more are called polypeptides. Hormones such as ACTH and vasopressin are important polypeptides.

Endorphins not only ease pain, but also seem to give people a feeling of well-being, happiness, even a "high" when they are released in abundance by the brain. Many of you may have heard of "runner's high," a feeling of mild euphoria that overtakes a person who is in excellent physical condition and who has run a long distance.

Endorphins are not only released by the brain to counter pain, but apparently as a kind of "reward" to a body that is being kept it peak physical condition.

Melatonin helps stimulate endorphin activity whether you are in good physical condition or not, and can improve your inner feeling of well-being enough to make you want to get your physical body back into peak performance condition.

It's amazing to think that still today, the most accepted method of helping people deal with stress is to give them tranquilizers, drugs that dampen the spirit and make the brain not less sensitive to stress, but merely less able to read it.

In the early 1980s, tranquilizers, such as Valium (diazepam) were the most frequently prescribed drugs in the world. Despite a 30% decline in the number of prescriptions written in the U.S. for benzodiazepines between 1975 and 1980, more than 5 million people were taking some form of them each year. Although they are useful for relief of temporary anxiety and insomnia, a National Academy of Sciences report warned in 1979 that they are not effective for periods longer than two weeks.

The minor tranquilizers are considered generally safe when taken alone, but taking substantial amounts of these substances at the same time as alcohol can lead to coma or even death. Long-term administration of larger than usual doses of the benzodiazepines can cause physical dependence, with typical withdrawal symptoms ranging from nightmares to convulsions when the drug intake is stopped.

Such "downers" as Valium, Xanex, and even Thorazine (a major tranquilizer) are prescribed to people who are high strung and stressed out. The result is not a person free from stress, but a doped, sluggish, bombed, sleepy individual who certainly seems more mellow on the outside — but on the inside, they have been drained of their vital life force, the vigor, energy and enthusiasm from which true happiness and balance comes.

Tranquilizers seem the logical choice for a person who is too "high." But there is a clear distinction between a good kind of high and a bad kind of high. **A good high** is characterized by positive energy, enthusiasm, even a "lust" for life, if you will. A man on a good high can't wait to get up in the morning to tackle the challenges that await him. He works hard, but still has energy left over for doing the things he loves to other than work, such as golf, building model rockets, hang gliding, or hiking. He has plenty of time and energy to make love to his wife and spend quality time with his children. After a long day of satisfying work, he sleeps well, and the next day he starts his wonderful life all over again.

A bad high is characterized by the stressed-out businessman who works 15 hours a day, smokes too many cigarettes, drinks 20 cups of coffee a day, and works like hell out of the fear of being fired or not being able to pay his mortgage. He does not so much as enjoy his work, as he does it because he has to. After work, he is a wasted mass of exhausted flesh. He needs a drink badly to dull his senses, to ease the roiling stress that has been exploding in his chest, stomach and mind all day. The bad high energy man does not sleep well. His mind chatters without end, and he cannot block out all the worries of the day of hell he just lived through and the next session in hell that he will wake up to in the morning. He generally does not have time for hobbies — or for his wife and children — whom most likely left him a long time ago because he was so impossible to live with.

Both the good high and the bad high enables people to get things done. Indeed, either one may be the company president. The only problem is that the bad high individual will have a heart attack or stroke at age 45, while the good high individual will work hard, play hard and enjoy life at a brisk level of activity for as long as what he is doing brings enjoyment and positive productivity. The bad high person cannot enjoy being president of the company because the climb to the top of that mountain has been an agonizing journey over a field of hot, broken glass — and he was barefoot all the way!

Melatonin can help just about anyone become the first guy, and stop being the second guy. That's because, unlike tranquilizers which only dull the pain, melatonin scrubs the pain from the chemical system of the human body, allowing you to undergo the stress of modern life, but not pay (at least) the physical price for it.

To be sure, there is more to all of this than taking a magic pill that will solve all your problems. Melatonin is not that magic pill — it is simply a powerful tool that gives us a fighting chance while we search deeper and make the changes in our life we need to be happier and healthier.

Melatonin is not going to counter the effects of too much drinking on a daily basis. It is not going to take back the cruel words you barked at your children or spouse. It is not going to drop a promotion into your lap without you having to do a single lick of work to earn it.

Rather, melatonin will help protect you from the bad things you do as much as it can, and will greatly bolster your conscious effort to make positive changes in your life to reduce stress.

Even for those people who, for whatever reason, cannot get a grip on their stress, melatonin may give them a bit more time and make them feel a bit less stressful than they otherwise might have been.

Melatonin and Cancer

Melatonin appears to slow the growth of cancerous tumors. In a British study on 14 cancer patients with cancers of different types, researchers found that melatonin can be extremely valuable in treating "untreatable" metastatic cancer patients, particularly in improving their quality of life. Moreover, based on its effects on the immune system, melatonin could be tested in association with other anti-tumor treatments. **The key is melatonin's effect on the immune system.** When the immune system is functioning properly, cancer does not have a chance to get started because as soon as an abnormal cell in the body is identified, the immune system sends a team over to bump it off.

That's why cancer is primarily a disease of old age. As people grow older, their immune systems stop working as efficiently as they did when they were young. The primary reason the immune system stops working is hormonal. Thus, bolstering the flagging hormone systems of elderly people may be the key to preventing millions of cases of cancer every year.

Melatonin appears able to play a key part in the entire process. Many doctors are currently experimenting with melatonin, giving it to cancer patients along with more traditional treatments, such as chemotherapy and radiation.

The results are extremely encouraging. These results include advanced cancer patients whose condition are considered either hopeless or so far advanced that nothing can bring them back from the edge of death. In addition to helping the body fight off the cancer itself, melatonin appears to strengthen the body against the negative side effects of chemotherapy and radiation, which damages the body's ability to fight off disease.

Is melatonin a cure for cancer? No. There is no indication that melatonin can erase cancer from a body completely, but it can give a person a fighting chance of recovery, a greater chance than they would have without it. Also, it may prevent cancer from developing in the first place in healthy people.

Melatonin and Alzheimer's Disease

We've talked about Alzheimer's a lot in previous chapters on estrogen, DHEA and testosterone, but melatonin has a key role to play as well in the battle against this dreaded disease of old age. New studies have found that people currently suffering from Alzheimer's have reduced levels of melatonin in their cerebrospinal fluid as compared to people of the same age who do not have Alzheimer's Disease. Because circadian rhythms are disrupted in Alzheimer's disease, it seems there is a direct link between melatonin levels and this disease.

Also, because melatonin is a so-called superhormone, meaning it effects and regulates a variety of other important hormones, bringing this substance back into balance with youthful parameters almost certainly has a major contribution to make in the ongoing battle against Alzheimer's and other forms of senile dementia.

Melatonin and Arthritis

Many clinical and experimental observations have suggested the existence of a relationship between melatonin, the pineal gland and so-called neoplastic diseases.

Interestingly, doctors have long observed a relationship between sleeping patterns and arthritis. People who can't seem to get a good night's sleep are more prone to arthritic conditions. When considering that melatonin helps a person get to sleep, it is not a big leap to look at melatonin imbalances as a possible culprit in the disease of arthritis. Also, once people develop arthritis, sleep is more difficult because of pain, stiffness and difficulty lying in bed, turning over, etc. Thus, melatonin's ability to aid sleep may help arthritic people rest better and feel better in the morning.

More than one researcher has reported about the effects of melatonin on neoplastic diseases and as a synchronizer of biological rhythms. One researcher used melatonin as a therapy against fibrosing diseases (particularly scleroderma) for several years, and the results were something to get excited about.

In a study conducted with people suffering from rheumatoid arthritis, melatonin was injected directly into the blood stream, and results were encouraging. Researchers observed significant improvements, both subjectively and objectively. Researchers caution, however, that these results are still to be considered preliminary, before a verification on a larger number of patients is performed.

The most commonly used dose has been of 10 mg injected directly into the body. Still, both lower and higher doses have proven effective in individual cases. A range comprised between 5 and 30 mg has proved compatible both with regard to the beneficial effects and to the absence of side effects.

As the starting material, a lyophilized product, available in vials or phials, containing the peptide and an inert excipient is used. At the time of use, the lyophilized product is diluted in water to produce an injectable solution, in proportion of 5 ml of water to every 10mg of melatonin. Patients with rheumatoid arthritis and serious articular diseases were selected. They expressly consented to the experiment. The knee joint was selected for experimental purposes.

The patients that underwent the melatonin injections had been examined before the test both with radiological methods and with an MR exam of specific affected joints. The clinical examination was done 3, 7, 15, and 30 days after treatment. A subsequent dose was injected monthly for three more months. Finally, a MR exam of the affected joint was performed.

Using a variety of measurement criteria, just about all the arthritis sufferers showed significant improvement — less pain, decreased swelling, greater range of movement — after direct injections of melatonin and water.

Lots more study needs to be done on injectable melatonin and arthritis patients, but the future looks promising for this kind of therapy.

Melatonin and Exposure to Electromagnetic Fields

Scientists have long known that sunlight is the No. 1 environmental influence involving the internal clock and the late-night burst in melatonin production which results. But sunlight may not be the only factor influencing melatonin production. There is some evidence that the earth's magnetic field may also be an environmental signal affecting circadian rhythms in humans. When shielded from the earth's ambient magnetic field, human circadian rhythms can become disrupted.

The phenomenon of terrestrial magnetism results from the fact that the entire earth behaves as an enormous magnet. The English physician and natural philosopher William Gilbert was the first to demonstrate this similarity in about 1600, although the effects of terrestrial magnetism had been utilized much earlier in primitive compasses.

The magnetic poles of the earth do not correspond with the geographic poles of its axis. The north magnetic pole is presently located off the western coast of Bathurst Island, in the Canadian Northwest Territories, almost 1290 km (almost 800 mi) northwest of Hudson Bay. The south magnetic pole is presently situated at the edge of the Antarctic continent in AdÈlie Land about 1930 km (about 1200 mi) northeast of Little America.

The position of the magnetic poles is not constant and shows an appreciable change from year to year. Variations in the magnetic field of the earth include secular variation, the change in the direction of the field caused by the shifting of the poles. This is a periodic variation that repeats itself after 960 years. A smaller annual variation also exists, as does a diurnal, or daily, variation that can be detected only by sensitive instruments.

Measurements of the secular variation show that the entire magnetic field has a tendency to drift westward at the rate of 19 to 24 km (12 to 15 mi) per year.

Intensity measurements are made with instruments called magnetometers, which determine the total intensity of the field and the intensities in the horizontal and vertical directions. The intensity of the magnetic field of the earth varies in different places on its surface. In the temperate zones it amounts to about 0.6 oersted, of which 0.2 oersted is in a horizontal direction.

Exposure to electromagnetic fields, which we'll call EMFs for short, by everything from household appliances to powerlines may be even more significant than previously though.

There have been documented cases of altered neural function from exposure to something called ELF, which stands for extremely low frequency fields, which are found near high-voltage powerlines. Included in altered brain functioning is a lowering of the amount of melatonin the brain produces. Thus, people living near power lines may benefit from taking melatonin supplements.

But there are other cases where too much melatonin production may be the problem. For example, EMFs have been blamed for a variety of effects including cancer, emotional depression, and disorientation. But by what means can EMF have these effects on people? One documented biological response to EMF is suppression of the normal nighttime increase in production of melatonin.

Because it is located at the base of the brain, the pineal gland may be extra sensitive to EMFs, just as the skin is sensitive to temperatures it comes into contact with.

The discovery of sensitivity to magnetic fields in mammals resulted from studies of migrating and homing animals by a researcher in Europe in 1980. These scientists were investigating how migrating animals, especially birds, are able to navigate over vast distances correctly. Many species of birds, for example, fly thousands of miles and return not only to the same area, but to the very same nest they occupied the previous season! They do so without the aid of modern technology, road maps or any other human contrivance. How do they get the job done? Finding the answer, as you will see, tells us something about melatonin in the brain and how it affects your life.

Scientists theorized that birds use the earth's magnetic field as a navigational clue. Researchers started by investigating the effects of a magnetic field on the electrophysiological activity of the pineal gland. In one experiment, they found that when they altered the direction of the magnetic field around guinea pigs there was a simultaneous change in electrical activity in their pineal cells while other brain areas showed no response.

When they exposed human volunteers to magnetic fields, they found that as the magnetic field was changed volunteers showed lowered blood melatonin concentrations. However, when they later attempted to repeat the experiment, they could find no effect on volunteers. This is an example of the difficulty researchers have frequently had in obtaining consistent results in EMF experiments.

After obtaining these results, researchers decided to examine the magnetic sensitivity of the pineal in birds to see if they could find more clues or connections between the pineal and EMFs. They found that the day/night relationship of the brain's response to melatonin was abolished when either the pineal gland was removed or when the magnetic field was changed—thus suggesting that the pineal is necessary for this daily rhythm and that magnetic fields can interfere with the pineal's function.

When scientists exposed pigeons to magnetic fields, they found the pineal gland was the most active area in the brain. Also, N-acetyltransferase (NAT), an enzyme involved in melatonin production, was reduced significantly by magnetic field exposure.

Other researchers found similar sensitivity to EMFs in rats. In experiments done in the 1980s, scientists exposed rats to electric fields for a month and studied the effects on melatonin and NAT. The normal nocturnal rise in melatonin levels was eliminated and the enzyme activity was likewise severely attenuated (see discussion of circadian biorhythms above).

When EMF exposure was discontinued, pineal melatonin returned to normal levels within three days. Scientists theorized that EMF exposure may suppress pineal melatonin by delaying production of

NAT. Apparently a small change in the activity of this enzyme was able to cause a large change in pineal production of melatonin.

Other researchers later confirmed pineal EMF sensitivity in rats. They found that when rats were exposed for a month to an electric field, the nighttime rise in melatonin was significantly reduced, but the amount of suppression was the same at all intensities of EMF exposure. In experiments done since, researchers have sometimes been able to confirm EMF inhibition of pineal function and at other times have not, due to factors which are not really understood. The EMF effect seems to depend on how carefully the experiment is done and, perhaps, on how much laboratory animals have adapted to our artificial, EMF-filled environment.

After such fascinating results with birds and rats, scientists were ready for experiments on humans.

To get started, they exposed human volunteers to EMF from electric blankets and then measured melatonin levels. Volunteers were given either specially modified electric blankets (which switched on and off twice as often and produced magnetic fields 50% stronger than conventional electric blankets), or conventional electric blankets, or traditional blankets. Volunteers used the blankets nightly for 7 weeks. While volunteers using conventional electric blankets demonstrated no differences from those who used traditional blankets, those in the group using the special high-EMF blankets had significantly lower nighttime melatonin levels. This experiment shows that low-frequency EMFs can depress night-time melatonin levels and suggests that interaction with the pineal is one possible mechanism by which EMF affects humans.

The most extensive and controversial studies with humans were done over a 12-year period by German scientists. They tested the influence of electric fields on circadian rhythms in a specially constructed underground building. Volunteers were unable to see the day/night cycles outside the unit so that their internal biorhythms were no longer circadian. Circadian rhythms are the internal biorhythms cued by the advent of day and night. When day and night cues are missing, the rhythms still occur but become independent of external cues and are referred to as "free-running" rhythms. Often the biological day length increases to 25 hours, becoming desynchronized with day and night cues.

Scientists found that individuals living in the shielded rooms without exposure to EMF exhibited longer free-running rhythms, larger variation in length of the rhythms, and increased desynchronization. In all the volunteers exposed to EMF, the length of free-running rhythms was shorter on average by one and one-fifth hours.

Interestingly, scientists found that when electric fields were switched on and off over a period of 5-7 days, many of the subjects' internal biorhythms synchronized to the field alterations so that biorhythms which had followed the rising and setting of the sun were now following the increase and decrease in the electric field.

Scientists found similar results in a series of experiments using finches, although other researchers have as yet been unable to duplicate the experiment, causing some scientists to doubt the original results.

Two illnesses which are held in check by normal pineal function are also suspected of being caused by exposure to EMF: cancer and emotional depression.

Melatonin treatment can inhibit the growth and metastasis of tumors in experimental animals. Administration of melatonin can also inhibit growth of several types of laboratory-grown cancer cells, and melatonin has a direct protective action against genetic damage.

Conversely, inactivation or removal of the pineal gland or inhibition of the release of melatonin has been shown to increase the rate of breast cancer in rats.

Evidence for a similar anticancer function for melatonin in humans is indirect. In blind women, melatonin production was found to be higher at all times and the incidence of breast cancer in these women was correspondingly lower. On the other hand, patients with breast or prostate cancer have lowered levels of melatonin, although it is not possible to say if this is a cause or effect. Melatonin has also been shown to have a stimulatory effect on immune function, which would give increased protection against cancer.

Psychological Effects

In addition, melatonin rhythms may be linked to psychological disorders. Several studies have suggested that disrupted circadian rhythms may contribute to affective disorders, emotional disturbances, and depressive reactions. Lowered levels of melatonin excretion have also been linked to seasonal depressive disorders.

Given this information, can we conclude that lower levels of melatonin caused by EMF exposure leave us more open to cancer and depression? There are over 50 epidemiologic studies which point to a moderately elevated cancer risk in children and adults exposed to EMF. Further, results from at least three studies have indicated an association between EMF exposure and depressive illness. In the most recent of the studies, suicide rates were increased in populations that lived near overhead transmission lines.

At the present time the direct evidence for EMF involvement in human disease is weak. However, experiments are now under way to:

1) measure melatonin levels in people exposed to EMF,

2) determine if EMF can reduce melatonin levels and by how much, and

3) correlate reduced melatonin levels with health effects like spontaneous abortion or cancer.

Our Magnetoreceptor?

The idea that animals respond to EMFs has experienced a slow but gradual increase in scientific interest. The ultimate goal of research mentioned here is identification of the physiological and anatomical components of a magnetoreceptor, an organ capable of sensing magnetic fields, and determining how EMFs can have an effect on people and animals. Once we know if the pineal really is the magnetoreceptor we will have a key to answer the question of how EMFs could be responsible for the variety of ills attributed to them.

When we can say, without a doubt, that exposure to EMF results in an inhibition of pineal melatonin in humans, we will have found a major piece of the puzzle of how EMF exposure could have an effect on our well-being. But the complete puzzle will still not be solved because it will then be necessary to find out how much of a decrease in melatonin is required to affect humans and whether or not exposure to EMF has the ability to decrease melatonin to that extent. Scientists still have their work cut out for them.

Dosage

We'll tell you more about how much melatonin each individual should take in the chapter on how to take hormones, but let's touch on dosage here.

But how much melatonin should you take? The appropriate dose can vary enormously from person to person. Some people fair well on a tiny 0.1 mg, while others need as much as 200 mg to bring about the results they are looking for. That's a whopping 2000-fold difference between the lowest dose and the highest!

Melatonin is available in a wide variety of doses, from .01 mg tablets to 3 mg tablets and some even higher. Many melatonin users have worked out a system by which they start taking 3 mg tablets at 11 p.m., and then adjust their dose from there, up or down. If they found that they slept well but were drowsy in the morning, they cut the dose in half. If they found the dose had little or no sleep-inducing effect, they increased the dose by 3 mg each night until they got the desired effect. Some people get good results from less than one milligram while many others land in the 20 mg per night range. Experience has shown, however, that the bulk of the population get the best results between 3 and 10 mg per night.

Precautions

Thus, proper timing may be crucial for the most effective use of melatonin. Individual differences in the absorption and metabolism of melatonin may account for the differences in size and timing of the resulting melatonin pulse. For example, doctors were treating a 36-year-old blind woman who was suffering from persistent sleeping problems. Her doctors reasoned that her blindness prevented sunlight from cuing her circadian rhythm, resulting in such bad daytime fatigue that she simply could not stay awake through an entire day. On the other hand, she was awake and restless all night, most of the time unable to sleep. Doctors needed a way to reset her biological clock without the help of good old sunlight. They tried melatonin. After two unsuccessful treatment regimens with 5 mg and 10 mg melatonin administered at about 10:30 p.m., doctors tried a third regimen of only 5 mg administered at 8 p.m. for three weeks. This approach resulted in a successful readjustment of the woman's sleep patterns and internal biological clock.

The woman's case illustrates the importance of not only adjusting the dosage but also the time of the dose. Timing is more important when taking melatonin than the other superhormones. For example, one long-time melatonin user recently gave himself a terrible day of jet lag-like symptoms — grogginess, fatigue, fuzzy thinking — by taking melatonin at 3 a.m. after staying up late one night. He thought it would be better than not taking it at all, but the next day he was fatigued and exhausted all day. He did not regain his normal balance until the next evening when he took his tablet at 10 p.m. The moral of the story is, taking melatonin relies strongly on timing. If you ignore this aspect of this superhormone, it will be impossible for you to realize the tremendous benefits it has for you.

NOTES

_____

_____

_____

_____

Chapter 8

How to Take
Youth Renewing Hormones

If you have read this far, you should be getting very excited about the possibilities which hormone replacement therapy holds for you.

But how to do it? How do you start yourself on a balanced program of super hormone replenishment safely? How do you know how much to take, and how often? Where do you find the hormones and other substances we have talked about in this book?

In this chapter, we will guide you through the process so that you can begin reaping the benefits of the youth-returning and youth enhancing power of hormone replacement therapy.

Fortunately, many of the hormones and other supplements you need can be found in any health food store. You can walk right in and simply choose what you need off the shelf, without need for a doctor's prescription.

Many of the other hormones we have talked about can be obtained only through a licensed doctor. But that's okay, because we DO NOT recommend you proceed with this plan of action without the careful supervision and advice of your physician. Also, you are going to need a doctor and the help of a modern medical lab to determine what your personal body chemistry is lacking, and what it already has plenty of. Each human being is different. Some lucky people maintain youthful hormone levels and balances of all the right stuff in their blood streams well into their 90s and 100s — that's why they live that long! Others, however, begin having problems as soon as they hit their early 40s. To find out where you stand, you need a thorough examination of your blood, the kind of test only a clinic or hospital with a modern medical lab is qualified to perform.

For Men:

For a healthy man, age 40 is the time to start visiting a doctor once a year for a complete medical check up. Even if you feel fine, your chances of contracting some kind of harmful medical condition increases dramatically as you reach age 40 and beyond.

Diseases of the prostate are of special concern for men. That's because more than 85 percent of all men will experience at least some kind of prostate problem at some time in their post-40 lifetime.

There are two primary concerns with the prostate. The first is called BPH, which stands for benign prostatic hyperplasia. This is a fancy way of saying enlargening of the prostate. After age 40, the prostate of most men begins to grow, and continues to grow until they die. For the majority of men, this may not be a problem, as long as no other disease is involved. However, for a significant percentage of men, BPH will lead to a variety of problems which include sexual dysfunction, urinary problems, infections of the urinary tract and bladder, and even kidney problems.

The second concern is cancer of the prostate, an extremely common form of cancer in older men. An additional danger of prostate cancer is the difficulty in detecting it. Prostate cancer can be present for years upon years before a man begins to feel any symptoms or any discomfort. Thus, a regular test called a PSA and also a DRE is highly recommended to check for signs of prostate cancer, giving doctors early warning on treatment options.

The three most common major prostate problems are:

(1) benign prostatic hypertrophy, most commonly called BPH

(2) prostate cancer

(3) prostatitis, which is a general term for a number of conditions, including bacterial and viral infections

In addition to prostate checks, men should have a CBC done, which is a complete blood count. They should also have their cholesterol levels checked (both HDL and LDL), and an annual chest X-ray is a good idea as well.

Other tests which round out the optimum physi-cal check-up for men:

- Blood sugar test
- Fecal blood occult test
- Baseline liver function test
- Thyroid function test
- A chest X-ray for TB
- A reading of all hormone levels

For women:

The big killer of women over the age of 40 is breast cancer. Thus, all women should perform regular self-examinations and have a mammogram once a year or every other year. Women should also have a gynecological examination, including a Pap smear and an examination for colon cancer. Also for women:

- A CBC, complete blood count
- Anemia test
- Cholesterol check
- Liver function test
- Test for diabetes
- Thyroid function test
- Fecal blood occult test
- Chest x-ray for TB

By the way, women who are pregnant should not take hormone supplements, unless specifically directed to do so by a doctor. Pregnancy is a time of great hormone manipulation in the female on behalf of Mother Nature. This is at least one time when it's best to let hormones take a "natural" course.

Taking DHEA

DHEA is easy to come by because you do not need a prescription from a medical doctor to get it. You can walk into any health food store and buy a bottle of your own right off the shelf. This is both good and bad. Good because you don't need the expense of both a doctor and pharmacist to obtain this valuable drug. It's bad because many people upon hearing about the fantastic benefits of DHEA may be tempted to go out, buy a large bottle of DHEA tablets, and start downing them like sugar cubes. Many people will not even check the dosage they have purchased, and will simply start popping one, two, or three pills a day.

Many people think that if a little bit will help, a lot will help even more. With any kind of drug or food supplement, this is almost never the case, and the same can be said for DHEA.

Before anyone begins to take DHEA, they should have their blood checked to get a true read-out of what their actual level of DHEA is. Normal DHEA levels for a 29 year old man is 3,600 nanoram per deciliter of plasma. For women, normal youthful levels are 2,600 nanograms per deciliter of plasma. If you are below these levels, it is probably a good idea for you to take DHEA. If you are not below those levels, there is little reason to raise your DHEA level even higher.

A blood test is not the only way to measure DHEA levels in your body. You may also undergo what is called a salivary hormone profile. In this simple test, a small amount of your saliva is sent to a lab where hormone levels in the sample are measured. Both the blood test and the saliva test are considered to be about equally accurate in determining hormone levels in the human body.

We are assuming that those of you getting your hormone levels checked are over the age of 40. For younger people, there is almost no chance you will be deficient in these vital hormone substances if you are otherwise in good physical condition. On the other hand, if you suspect you are not in optimum health, you should see your doctor for a check-up and at that time you can ask to have your DHEA levels tested.

If you are over 40, and indeed you find low levels of DHEA, you may want to start with a dose of between 25 and 50 milligrams per day, or every other day. Many doctors recommend starting your intake every other day. Other doctors say taking DHEA every other day is also a good idea because, in some people, artificial intake of DHEA can "fool" the body into stopping production of its own natural DHEA. The brain may read the blood level of DHEA in your body and think: "Well, it's already high. No need to make the adrenal glands produce more!"

Most people at age 40 have half the level of DHEA that they had when they were 20, although individuals vary widely. Once again, it depends on what your blood levels show. Also, those of you who are at the low end of DHEA loss may need only the 25 mg tablet every other day, while those of you seriously low may be better off with the 50 mg dosage.

An important note: it is best to take DHEA in the morning because that is the time of day your body naturally produces this substance.

Have your blood checked after a month of taking either 25 or 50 mg of DHEA every other day. At this time, your doctor may recommend a change in dosage, depending on what your new read-out is. Your doctor may want to see you again in another month. Once your doctor is satisfied that you have found the right dosage and that your DHEA level is at normal levels for a youthful person, you should have the level checked every six months.

For those of you taking drugs to counter other conditions, such as high cholesterol or diabetes, your new adjustment or your hormone level may be altering the need for these other drugs. DHEA, for example, has been shown to reduce cholesterol levels dramatically in some people. Thus, you need to look at all the parameters. If you no longer need drugs for cholesterol as a result of taking DHEA, your doctor would want to know about it. Again, this points again to the importance of working closely with a doctor to keep tabs on all aspects of your blood chemistry and health.

Another important note: If you are buying DHEA over the counter, make sure that what you are getting is true DHEA. Some manufacturers sell products which purportedly change to DHEA after it gets into your body. You will find such information on the fine print somewhere on the bottle. This is not the kind you want to buy. Rather, you want DHEA that clearly states it is pharmaceutical-grade DHEA, meaning it is some 99 percent pure. If you are unsure about which DHEA is which, ask the owner of the health food store for help.

DHEA comes in many different forms, including skin creams, eye drops, gels, time release pills, or micro-doses, which are very small doses of DHEA. Again, ask your doctor or a pharmacist which is best for you in your current situation. Remember that rubbing DHEA cream on your skin has the same ultimate effect of swallowing DHEA tablets. With the skin cream, the DHEA is absorbed through the skin. Many people take a DHEA tablet, and also use DHEA skin cream to get rid of wrinkles, blemishes, or whatever, not realizing that the skin cream is increasing the total overall dosage.

Pregnenolone

Pregnenolone is sold over the counter like DHEA is. You do not need a doctor's prescription to obtain this hormone. Once again, that should not give anyone license to simply start downing the stuff like popcorn. You should only take this hormone while following a sensible program guided by a doctor.

As we said in the chapter devoted to pregnenolone in this book, natural levels of this hormone begin to decline dramatically in people once they reach the age of 45. By the time age 75 rolls around, we have some 60 to 70 percent less pregnenolone in our body compared to age 29. **Once again you need a blood test to find out what your current level is. Once again, either a blood test or a saliva test will tell the story.**

Many people who are low on pregnenolone will find that they are not as clear headed and as mentally sharp as they used to be. Those who begin taking pregnenolone usually see results within just a few hours of swallowing their first tablet. They begin to feel more clear headed. The other benefits of pregnenolone take longer to make themselves known. For example, arthritics may not see immediate results, but after a month or two, arthritis may lessen considerably or even disappear for some people. Also, as we have said elsewhere, pregnenolone is many times safer than most medications for arthritis, with side effects that are nonexistent.

Testosterone for Men

Testosterone is available only through a doctor's prescription, but you should not let this stop you from seeing your doctor and getting your testosterone level checked.

Most men see a significant decline in testosterone production at around age 50. One of the first signs of a dwindling testosterone count is a loss of interest in sex. A loss of energy is also a symptom, as is a loss in muscle tone, muddled thinking and other signs.

Testosterone is more complex to test accurately since a lab technicians must check for both testosterone and free or unbound testosterone. You must have adequate amounts of unbound testosterone to have the levels you need to feel "like yourself."

Most doctors do not recommend taking testosterone orally because it has been shown to contribute to possible liver cancer. Rather, an injection is best. You blood test will determine which dosage is best. A common injection is 200 mg. Studies show testosterone injections are the most effective way to supplement the body with this substance, although it is common for many men to experience the greatest benefit after the first week of injection, with declining benefits until the next. This problem may be solved by the patch — a round, testosterone delivery system which men wear on their skin. It is worn on the back or on the butt. It delivers a steady flow on testosterone into the system, making the effect less radical than the up and down feeling many men get with spaced injections.

Testosterone also comes in creams and gels to be used as a skin cream, and as a sublingual tablet which dissolves under the tongue. The advantage of the latter is the fact that, taken this way, testosterone is absorbed directly into the blood stream, bypassing the liver, a potential problem for cancer with some forms of testosterone supplement.

All men must have a complete physical check-up before beginning testosterone therapy. It is especially important to check for prostate cancer, which means both a digital rectal exam (DRE) and a PSA test, which stands for prostate specific antigen. And because testosterone increases the red blood cell count, frequent checks should be made to make sure the count does not get too high.

Testosterone for Women

Yes, women also need this so-called male hormone, and if the body stops producing it naturally, testosterone supplement may be called for. Interestingly, loss of sex drive in women is also a sign of low testosterone levels.

As you might expect, women should receive a lot less testosterone supplement than men. Again, a blood test will tell the story of what each woman may or may not need. Like men, women should also avoid pill form testosterone in favor of a shot or what are known as skin pellets, which doctors implant under the skin. Drug companies are not yet producing skin patches for women, and the current patches deliver too high a dose for women. Women who are given testosterone should have regular blood checks to monitor their level of testosterone to maintain optimum levels.

Estrogen

A lot is known about estrogen because doctors have prescribed it millions upon millions of times to women all around the world, mostly to treat menopause. You cannot buy estrogen over the counter. You can only obtain it through a doctor's prescription.

The most common form of estrogen, Premarin, which we discussed in the estrogen chapter, is extracted from the urine of pregnant animals, most often a horse. Premarin is prescribed so often it actually wins the prize as the No.1 prescribed drug in America. Because doctors are so familiar with it, they are comfortable in prescribing it. Doctors love known quantities. They don't like surprises. Premarin has been around so long, it offers little in the way of problems which any good doctor does not know how to handle.

Many doctors, however, are beginning to favor another form of estrogen called Estrace (estradiol) over Premarin because the former is more closely matched to the kind of estrogen actually produced by the human body. Another advantage Estrace has over Premarin is that it can be made into a variety of dosages, whereas Premarin comes in only one size — .625 mg pills.

Estrogen is now available in skin patches as well. It is worn on the stomach or posterior. It needs only to be changed twice a week. Many doctors are beginning to prefer the patch as the best hormone delivery system because it sends estrogen directly into the blood stream, avoiding the liver where estrogen can create side effect problems. Also, the patch does not contribute to high blood pressure or abnormal blood clotting as some other forms of estrogen have been shown to do to a certain percentage of women.

Estrogen comes in creams and gels. Estrogen cream applied directly to the vagina helps ease vaginal drying and other problems.

No matter what kind of estrogen you use, or what delivery system is used, blood levels should be checked periodically so that your doctor can determine that your are getting the level you should be getting. Also, women must be sure to have a breast exam to look for cancerous lumps. Estrogen can stimulate the growth of existing breast lumps, although it will not promote the growth of new lumps. In fact, estrogen has been shown to prevent the formation of other cancers in the body, especially colon cancer.

Of course, women who are taking estrogen should consider its close companion, progesterone. So let's discuss this very important hormone right now.

Progesterone

This hormone works closely with estrogen. Without progesterone, it is difficult to maintain safe levels of a variety of hormones in the female body. For one thing, it prevents a condition called hyperplasia, which is a thickening of the lining of the uterus. Such a condition can lead to uterine cancer.

You need a prescription from a doctor to obtain progesterone. The most common form of this hormone is marketed under then name Provera. It comes in 5 mg and 10 mg doses, which is taken for 10 to 14 days out of each month.

We should point out that there is a difference between Provera and what is called natural progesterone. Natural progesterone is also only available only prescription from your doctor. Many doctors prefer this form of progesterone because it has fewer side effects than Provera, which can cause mood swings, headaches and bloating. Natural progesterone produces none of these in most women, and in fact, can make women feel even better than they do without it.

Doctors will prescribe progesterone to you if they feel you need it after a careful examination of your blood levels and by taking careful note of how you feel and what your symptoms are. Your blood levels will be checked periodically to make sure all levels are within proper readings considered safe and normal.

Thyroid Hormone

A lack of thyroid hormone is most often associated with extreme daily fatigue. Thyroid hormone is the substance which provides fuel to just about every cell in the human body. Mental confusion and loss of memory are also telling symptoms of low thyroid hormone, as is increased sensitivity to cold. People with low thyroid levels feel reenergized and wonderfully clear headed after a doctor helps them bring their thyroid hormone levels back into balance.

Thyroid hormone levels decline with age, as do most of the other hormone levels. Some people are more lucky than others. Thyroid hormone levels can decline at any age for people with specific thyroid problems. A doctor will use a blood test to determine if your thyroid is functioning properly. That means looking at all the different kinds of thyroid hormone, including T3, T4 and TSH, all of which we talked about in the chapter on thyroid hormone.

An easy way you can check for thyroid hormone deficiency is to take your basal temperature. You do this by simply placing a thermometer under your arm in the morning and before you get out of bed. Leave it there for 10 minutes. If the temperature falls below 97.4 degrees Fahrenheit, you may have a thyroid hormone deficiency.

You cannot buy this substance at a health food store. You must see your doctor for a prescription. The proper dosage may be difficult to determine at first. Get too much and you will feel agitated and irritable, and you may even experience a fluttering heart. If this is the case, get yourself to a doctor as soon as possible for further treatment. On the other hand, if you take too little thyroid hormone, it will not solve your problems. Close work with your doctor will find the proper dose for you. Each person is an individual requiring individual treatment. It's best to follow the advice of your doctor closely when taking this drug.

Human growth hormone

The good thing about human growth hormone is that not everyone will need to take this as a supplement, in fact, most will not. The bad news about it is the fact that it is tremendously expensive — up to $20,000 per year. If you don't have good insurance, you will have a tough time affording this drug. Even if you have insurance, your co-payment is likely to be hefty, depending on your policy.

Human growth hormone is available only through a doctor's prescription. A doctor usually prescribes it for specific conditions, such as kidney problems, heart problems, or for a class of ailments called wasting syndromes, which may have various causes, but all of which may be remedied with human growth hormone.

People who are prescribed to take this substance are usually given syringes which they inject into themselves at home. The syringes are premeasured and the usual prescription is for twelve doses over a period of 12 days. Most take a shot in the morning and another at night.

Again, injections of human growth hormone are used only in extreme cases. But that doesn't mean you can't increase your level of human growth hormone without the help of a doctor and without worry about any side effects. How on earth do you do that? Simply by taking up regular exercise. Doing so causes your body to increase its natural production of the stuff, providing you with all the benefits that come along with it. This is why many elderly people who get off their chairs and away from their televisions to take up some regular form of exercise see all kinds of rejuvenating effects on all aspects of their health. Not only do muscles grow stronger, but mental acuity returns and a general feeling of overall health and youthfulness returns.

Also, taking extremely safe hormones, such as DHEA, melatonin, pregnenolone, estrogen and testosterone can result in greater synthesis of human growth hormone in the body. So there are two ways to gain the advantages of HGH — through good old exercise and through a regimen of the other hormones we have spent a good part of this book speaking about.

Melatonin

Melatonin, which many medical experts think is the "hormone of hormones" because it acts as a regulator of many of the other hormones, is readily available in any health food store. You do not need a doctor's prescription to obtain this powerful hormone.

Few supplements have enjoyed a greater media honeymoon than has melatonin in the past two or three years. Some medical doctors go as far as saying that melatonin can keep people in a state of physical and mental youth no matter what their age — up to probably a limit of 120 years, or so. In studies with animals, melatonin has all but proved it can halt the aging process in it tracks and even reverse the effects of aging.

But how much melatonin should you take? The appropriate dose can vary enormously from person to person. Some people fair well on a tiny 0.1 mg, while others need as much as 200 mg to bring about the results they are looking for. That's a whopping 2000-fold difference between the lowest dose and the highest!

Melatonin is available in a wide variety of doses, from .01 mg tablets to 3 mg tablets and some even higher. Many melatonin users have worked out a system by which they start taking 3 mg tablets at 11 p.m., and then adjust their dose from there, up or down. If they found that they slept well but were drowsy in the morning, they cut the dose in half. If they found the dose had little or no sleep-inducing effect, they increased the dose by 3 mg each night until they got the desired effect. Some people get good results from less than one milligram while many others land in the 20 mg per night range. Experience has shown, however, that the bulk of the population get the best results between 3 and 10 mg per night.

Timing Is Important

An amazing amount of people make the mistake of taking melatonin during the day, only to find they become so drowsy the only thing they can think about is a good long nap! Do not take melatonin during the daytime hours when you are supposed to be up and alert! Take it before you go to bed — but not too late at night.

Thus, proper timing may be crucial for the most effective use of melatonin. Individual differences in the absorption and metabolism of melatonin may account for the differences in size and timing of the resulting melatonin pulse. For examples, doctors were treating a 36-year-old blind woman who was suffering from persistent sleeping problems. Her doctors reasoned that her blindness prevented sunlight from cuing her circadian rhythm, resulting in such bad daytime fatigue that she simply could not stay awake through an entire day. On the other hand, she was awake and restless all night, most of the time unable to sleep. Doctors needed a way to reset her biological clock without the help of good old sunlight. They tried melatonin. After two unsuccessful treatment regimens with 5 mg and 10 mg melatonin administered at about 10:30 p.m., doctors tried a third regimen of only 5 mg administered at 8 p.m. for three weeks. This approach resulted in a successful readjustment of the woman's sleep patterns and internal biological clock.

The woman's case illustrates the importance of not only adjusting the dosage but also the time of the dose. Timing is more important when taking melatonin than the other superhormones. For example, one long-time melatonin user recently gave himself a terrible day of jet lag-like symptoms — grogginess, fatigue, fuzzy thinking — by taking melatonin at 3 a.m. after staying up late on night. He thought it would be better than not taking it at all, but the next day he was fatigued and exhausted all day. He did not regain his normal balance until the next evening when he took his tablet at 10 p.m. The moral of the story is, taking melatonin relies strongly on timing. If you ignore this aspect of this superhormone, it will be impossible for you to realize the tremendous benefits it has for you.

Melatonin for Jet Lag

Even people who are young and who enjoy naturally high levels of melatonin production in their bodies can benefit from taking melatonin as a way to reset their biological clocks when they are thrown off by jet travel to different time zones. By now, hardly a single doctor in the world would disagree that melatonin is the best and only cure for jet lag.

All you have to do to reset your time clock is take 3 to 5 mg of melatonin prior to bedtime in your new destination. The next day, you will not suffer from ordinary jet lag, and rather, you should feel rested and refreshed as if you have had a normal day's sleep in your own bed in your own time zone. It is a good idea to continue your melatonin intake before bedtime each day of your new destination. When you return, you may have the same problem again — now your clock is not set for your own time zone. You remedy the situation by again taking 3 to 5 mg at bedtime until you feel you are back in the swing of your normal sleep-awake pattern.

Sleep Disorders

Melatonin may be the best medical news of the decade for people suffering from problems with sleeping. Thousands of people who otherwise cannot get to sleep at night are finding that rest comes easily if they tale 3 to 5 mg of melatonin before bedtime. The great thing about melatonin is that it helps people get to sleep without drugging them, disturbing their dream patterns, and without leaving them drowsy in the morning. Yes, melatonin can cause drowsiness if too large a dose is taken, but correcting the problem is as easy as reducing the dosage until you can fall asleep easily while waking up fresh and rested in the morning. Each individual will very likely have to do a bit of experimenting to find a dose that works best for them. Increase your dosage by 1 mg per night. You should fall comfortably asleep within a half hour of your chosen melatonin dosage.

If it takes longer to get to sleep, you most likely can handle a bigger dosage.

After two weeks of melatonin-induced sleep, you may find that you will be able to stop taking the hormone because your natural clock will have been reset, and you should continue to sleep normally. If your sleeplessness returns, go back to the melatonin. There are no known side-effects to taking melatonin over a long period of time, and it is without a doubt safer than taking other prescription or over-the-counter sleeping pills.

One last thing: The older you are, the more likely you will need a larger daily dose of melatonin. Ultimately, you should have a long talk with your doctor on what your particular dose should be. As with all the other hormones, you should have your level of melatonin tested by a professional medical lab. Be warned that anyone taking antidepressant drugs, antihistamines or antihypertensives should not take melatonin before talking it over with a doctor.

That's It!

It's true that taking advantage of the youth renewal properties of the hormones we have described in this chapter and in this book is not as easy as walking down to the local health food store and popping a few pills.

Because of this, many of you will simply give up and not implement the very program you need to possibly extend your lifespan by 30, 40 or 50 years.

We want to suggest to you that some extra effort will pay off big — what could be bigger than almost doubling your lifespan?

Yes, you may have to do a bit of leg work, have more than one visit to a doctor, endure a complete physical and a pin prick or three for blood tests, and such, but the end result will be an entirely new life — and longer life — for those of you who take the time to do thing right.

Have your levels of the eight essential hormones checked, and restore them to their proper balance, and you'll experience the return of nothing less than blissful youth and everything that comes with it — strength, sex drive, enthusiasm, endless energy — and that should be all the motivation you need.

NOTES

_____

_____

_____

_____

_____

_____

_____

Chapter 9

The Cutting Edge of Anti-aging Research

This is perhaps the most exciting chapter of this book. That's because we are going to examine the very cutting edge of medical technology and research as it applies to the process of aging, and the promise that technology may someday be able to not only stop the aging process completely, but reverse it for people who have already grown old.

We've already spoken quite a bit in previous chapters about something called free radicals, what they do to the human body, and why they are the focus of intense interest by anti-aging researchers around the world.

Also, we have seen that superhormones, such as DHEA, melatonin and others may be extremely effective substances for getting rid of free radicals in the human body. More research is needed to understand the full role of hormones in "scrubbing" free radicals.

The Vitamin Factor

But the good news is that a lot more detailed research has already been done on more familiar substances and their effects on free radicals — good old vitamins, specifically vitamins A, E, C and beta carotene. These are coming to be known as the "Big 4" in the battle against aging — primarily because of their apparent action against free radicals.

The Glucose Factor

Also in this chapter, we are going to examine another area in the study of aging which has to do with sugar — not the kind you eat, but the kind that exists in the blood. This kind of blood sugar is called glucose. Apparently, as people grow older, a process involving glucose and the breakdown of cell structure in the human body begins to accelerate. Scientists are learning more about this glucose aging factor, and we'll see if anything can be done about it.

Heat Shock Proteins

A third area of anti-aging research we are going to look at goes by the unusual name of "heat shock proteins, or HSPs for short. These are substances produced in the human body when cells are exposed to various stresses, such as excessive heat.

But heat is not the only factor that can trigger the development of HSPs. They can also be produced by exposure to toxic substances such as heavy metals and chemicals and even by behavioral and psychological stress. We'll find out what you can do about HSPs, and how avoiding them can help keep you young.

Genetics and DNA

This is perhaps the most promising area of research on the effort to find a true Fountain of Youth. Scientists are working diligently at unlocking the secrets of the most fundamental building blocks of the human body — the genes and what they are made up of — DNA, which stands for deoxyribonucleic acid. There are actually two kinds of these nucleic acids. The other is RNA, which stands for ribonucleic acid.

We'll tell you more about both of them and how they present exciting frontiers on the cutting edge of aging research.

The Theory of Free Radicals

First, let's look more closely at free radicals and then at how the Big 4 vitamins can help in getting rid of these little youth robbers from your body.

The free radical theory of aging, first proposed by Denham Harman at the University of Nebraska, says that damage caused by oxygen radicals is responsible for many of the bodily changes that come with aging.

Free radicals have been implicated not only in aging but also in degenerative disorders, including cancer, atherosclerosis, cataracts, and neurodegeneration.

A free radical is a molecule with an unpaired, highly reactive electron, An oxygen-free radical They damage cells and is a byproduct of normal metabolism, produced as may cause tissues and cells turn food and oxygen into energy. organs to age.

In need of a mate for its lone electron, the free radical takes an electron from another molecule, which in turn becomes unstable and combines readily with other molecules. A chain reaction can ensue, resulting in a series of compounds, some of which are harmful. They damage proteins, membranes, and nucleic acids, particularly DNA, including the DNA in mitochondria, the organelles within the cell that produce energy.

But free radicals do not go unchecked. Mounted against them is a multilayer defense system manned by anti oxidants that react with and disarm these damaging molecules. Anti oxidants include nutrients — the familiar vitamins C and E and beta carotene — as well as enzymes, such as superoxide dismutase (SOD), catalase, and glutathione peroxidase.

They prevent most, but not all, oxidative damage. Little by little the damage mounts and contributes, so the theory goes, to deteriorating tissues and organs. Support for the free radical theory comes from studies of anti oxidants, particularly SOD. SOD converts oxygen radicals into the also harmful hydrogen peroxide, which is then degraded by another enzyme, catalase, to oxygen and water.

Take Your Vitamins!

What all this means is that, to ward off premature aging, you must increase your daily intake of vitamins C, E, A and beta carotene! While some researchers are still unconvinced that these vitamins will actually scrub free radicals from the body, even the most skeptical scientists will admit that there is a lot of compelling circumstantial evidence — and some evidence better than circumstantial — that these four vitamins do, in fact, slow the aging process. Furthermore, it is almost certainly harmless to increase your intake of each of these vitamin by some 200 percent. They are also relatively inexpensive. You don't even have to buy bottled supplements. Increasing your intake of foods that contain these high levels of these vitamins will have the same if not better effect as bottled supplements.

While it is almost impossible to overdose on vitamin C (because it is essentially a food and your body processes it as such), large doses of vitamins E and A can produce toxic side effects in some people. Because of the ease, availability and low cost of increasing your vitamin C, E and A intake, it is one of the best things you can do right now to take a swat at the old Grim Reaper.

Another important point: Although vitamin C supplements are okay, most researchers agree that it's best to get your C directly from foods rich in the substance. **Here are the best sources of vitamin C:**

Broccoli	**Brussels sprouts**
Cabbage	**Cantaloupe**
Cauliflower	**Collard greens**
Grapefruit	**Grapefruit juice**

Oranges	Orange juice
Pineapple	Pineapple juice
Spinach	Strawberries

And many others, but the above have the highest concentration of vitamin C. Of course, many common fruits and vegetables have vitamin C and will be well worth including in your diet.

The best source of vitamin A other than supplements are:

Dried apricots	Cherries
Dandelions	Mangos
Sorrel	Cantaloupe
Carrots	Nectarines
Seaweeds	Papaya
Collard greens	Peaches
Kale	Prunes
Hot red peppers	Broccoli

The best sources of vitamin E other than supplements are:

Blackberries	Asparagus
Pears	Beet greens
Sesame Seeds	Broccoli
Sunflower Seeds	Brussel Sprouts
Almonds	Corn
Brazil Nuts	Leeks
Filberts	Spinach
Walnuts	Sweet potatoes

The best sources for beta carotene other than supplements are:

Beets	Spinach
Broccoli	Sweet potatoes
Butternut squash	Tomatoes
Carrots	Chicory greens
Kale	Watercress
Parsnips	Dandelions
Pumpkins	Mustard
Cantaloupe	Papaya
Milk	

Gerbils and Worms

A boost for the hypothesis that high levels of anti-oxidants can slow the aging process comes from a study of N-tert-butyl-alpha-phenylnitrone or PBN in gerbils. Although it does not occur naturally in the body, PBN works in much the same way as beta-carotene and other anti oxidants by binding and neutralizing free radicals.

Older gerbils had been shown to have increased levels of oxidized protein in their brains by two researchers, Robert A. Floyd at the Oklahoma Medical Research Foundation and John M. Carney at the University of Kentucky. Curious about the effects of anti-oxidants in older animals, Floyd and Carney designed an experiment to learn whether PBN could lower oxidized protein levels in gerbils' brains. Over a period of 14 days they gave PBN to two groups of gerbils, one made up of young adults, the other of older adults.

As the older gerbils were treated with PBN, their levels of oxidized protein decreased until they were nearly comparable to levels found in the younger animals. After treatment ended, oxidized protein gradually returned to pretreatment levels. PBN had no effect on the young gerbils.

While it is only one study and more are needed, this investigation supports the idea that maintaining anti oxidant defense levels may be critical during aging. It also suggests that an intervention such as PBN may someday provide the means.

Discovery of a mutant gene involved in the regulation of longevity of a primitive worm, C. elegans, may provide a clue as to how humans age. Normal development and longevity in the worm C. elegans are regulated by the age-1 gene. Lack of age-1 activity in adult worms, due to mutations in the age-1 gene, results in a doubling of adult life span. The research team of Drs. Gary Ruvkun, Jason Morris, and Heidi Tissenbaum at Massachusetts General Hospital/Harvard Medical School isolated and determined the DNA sequence of the normal and four mutant forms of the C. elegans age-1 gene. Further analysis revealed that the normal age-1 gene encodes the worm homolog of the enzyme phosphotidyl-inositol-3-OH-kinase (PI(3)K), a key biological mediator of cellular communication and signal transduction.

Analysis of animals with several different mutations in the age-1 gene showed that the age-1 PI(3)K protein functions specifically in the longevity pathway in C. elegans. The authors speculate that lower levels of PI(3)K activity may trigger a biochemical program in the worm, ultimately leading to a decreased rate of aging and senescence. However, they caution that it is not yet known whether phosphotidylinositol-mediated control of longevity is confined to C. elegans or is more generally applicable to regulation of aging and longevity in mammalian species including humans.

More Than a Human Phenomenon

Anti-aging researchers have also found that SOD levels are directly related to life span in 20 different species; longer-lived animals have higher levels of SOD, suggesting that the ability to fight free radicals has something to do with longer life spans. Levels of other anti oxidants — vitamin E and beta-carotene, for example — have also been correlated with life span.

Other studies have shown that inserting extra copies of the SOD gene into fruit flies extends their average life span. In three different laboratories, researchers have reported that transgenic fruit flies, carrying extra copies of the gene for SOD, live 5 to 10 percent longer than average.

Other experimental evidence lends support to the free radical hypothesis. For example, higher levels of SOD and catalase have been found in long-lived nematodes. And in another important study, giving gerbils a synthetic anti oxidant has reduced high levels of oxidized protein, a sign of aging, in their brains.

Glucose Crosslinking

Another suspect in cellular deterioration is blood sugar or glucose. In a process called non-enzymatic glycosylation or glycation, glucose molecules attach themselves to proteins, setting in motion a chain of chemical reactions that ends in the proteins binding together or crosslinking, thus altering their biological and structural roles. The process is slow but increases with time.

Crosslinks, which have been termed advanced glycosylation end products (AGEs), seem to toughen tissues and may cause some of the deterioration associated with aging. AGEs have been linked to stiffening connective tissue (collagen), hardened arteries, clouded eyes, loss of nerve function, and less efficient kidneys.

These are deficiencies that often accompany aging. They also appear at younger ages in people with diabetes, who have high glucose levels. Diabetes, in fact, is sometimes considered an accelerated model of aging. Not only do its complications mimic the physiologic changes that can accompany old age, but its victims have shorter-than-average life expectancies. As a result, much research on crosslinking has focused on its relationship to diabetes as well as aging.

One happy finding is that the body has its own defense system against crosslinking. Just as it has anti-oxidants to fight free-radical damage, it has other guardians, immune system cells called macrophages, that combat glycation. Macrophages with special receptors for AGEs seek them out, engulf them, break them down, and eject them into the blood stream where they are filtered out by the kidneys and eliminated in urine.

The only apparent drawback to this defense system is that it is not complete and levels of AGEs increase steadily with age. One reason is Glucose, the that kidney function tends to decline with fundamental source of advancing age. Another is that macrophages, like energy, react with and certain other components of the immune system, crosslinks essential become less active. Why is not known, but molecules. immunologists are beginning to learn more about how the immune system affects and is affected by aging. And in the meantime, diabetes researchers are investigating drugs that could supplement the body's natural defenses by blocking AGE formation.

Crosslinking interests gerontologists for several reasons. It is associated with disorders that are common among older people, such as diabetes; it progresses with age; and AGEs are potential targets for anti-aging drugs.

In addition, crosslinking may play a role in damage to DNA, which has become another important focus for research on aging.

Genetics

In laboratories all over the world, scientists are isolating specific genes, cloning them, mapping them to chromosomes, and studying their products to learn what they do and how they influence aging, and the possibility all this holds for making everyone stay young for a very long time.

As we have said previously, the human body seems to have a maximum life span of 120 to 130 years. Life span is different for different animals. Some turtles live for hundreds of years, while a dog or cat would be lucky to live 20 years.

Why? Scientists know part of the answer. What underlies these differences among species are genes, the coded segments of DNA strung like beads along the chromosomes of nearly every living cell. In humans, the nucleus of each cell holds 23 pairs of chromosomes, and together these chromosomes contain about 100,000 genes.

Before we go further, some background information about DNA will be helpful in understanding the discussion which follows.

The two classes of nucleic acids are the acids (DNA) and the ribonucleic acids (RNA). The backbones of both DNA and RNA molecules are shaped like helical strands. Their molecular weights are in the millions. To the backbones are connected a great number of smaller molecules of four different types.

The sequence of these molecules on the strand determines the code of the particular nucleic acid. This code, in turn, signals the cell how to reproduce either a duplicate of itself or the proteins it requires for survival.

All living cells contain the genetic material DNA. The cells of bacteria may have but one strand of DNA, but such a strand contains all the information needed by the cell in order to reproduce an identical offspring. The cells of mammals contain scores of DNA strands grouped together in chromosomes. In short, the structure of a DNA molecule or a combination of DNA molecules determines the shape, form, and function of the offspring. Some viruses, called retroviruses, contain only RNA rather than DNA, but viruses themselves are generally not considered true living organisms.

The pioneering research that revealed the general structure of DNA was performed by Francis Crick, James Dewey Watson, and Maurice Wilkins. Wilkins obtained an X-ray diffraction picture of the DNA molecule in 1951. Using this picture, Crick and Watson were able to construct a model of the DNA molecule that was completed in 1953. For their work, they received the 1962 Nobel Prize in physiology or medicine. Arthur Kornberg synthesized DNA from off-the-shelf substances, for which he was awarded, with Severo Ochoa, the 1959 Nobel Prize in physiology or medicine. The DNA that he synthesized, although structurally similar to natural DNA, was not biologically active. In 1967, however, Kornberg and a team of researchers at Stanford University succeeded in producing biologically active DNA from relatively simple chemicals.

Certain kinds of RNA have a slightly different function from that of DNA. They take part in the actual synthesis of the proteins a cell produces. This is of particular interest to virologists because many viruses reproduce by "forcing" the host cells to manufacture more viruses. The virus injects its own RNA into the host cell, and the host cell obeys the code of the invading RNA rather than that of its own. Thus the cell produces proteins that are, in fact, viruses instead of the proteins required for cell function. The host cell is destroyed, and the newly formed viruses are free to inject their RNA into other host cells.

The structure of two types of RNA and their function in protein production have been determined, one type by a team of Cornell University and U.S. Department of Agriculture investigators led by Robert W. Holley of Cornell, and the other type by James T. Madison and George A. Everet of the Department of Agriculture. Important research into the interpretation of the genetic code and its role in protein synthesis was also performed by the Indian-born American chemist Har Gobind Khorana at the University of Wisconsin Enzyme Institute and the American biochemist Marshall W. Nirenberg of the National Heart Institute. In 1970 Khorana achieved the first complete synthesis of a gene and repeated his feat in 1973. Since then one type of RNA has been synthesized. Also, in the early 1980s, a team of biologists at the National Jewish Hospital in Denver, Colorado, proved that in some cases RNA can function as a true catalyst.

Genes and Life Span

The link between genes and life span is unquestioned. The simple observation that some species live longer than others — humans longer than dogs, tortoises longer than mice — is one convincing piece of evidence. Another comes from recent, dramatic laboratory studies in which researchers, through selective breeding or genetic engineering, have been able to raise animals with extended life spans. For example, fruit flies bred selectively have lived nearly twice as long as average (see In the Lab of the Long-Lived Fruit Flies).

Longevity Genes

By demonstrating that genes are linked to life span, the long-lived fruit flies have set the stage for more questions. What specific genes are involved? What activates them? How do they influence aging and longevity? In numerous laboratories, the search for answers is on.

Some leads are coming from yeast cells in which researchers have found evidence of 14 genes that seem to be related to aging. Longevity-related genes have also been found in tiny worms called nematodes and in fruit flies. Like yeast, nematodes and fruit flies have short life spans and their genes, which are known and do not vary greatly, are relatively easy to study.

In the Lab of the Long-Lived Fruit Flies

A laboratory at the University of California, Irvine, is the home of thousands of Drosophila melanogaster or fruit flies that routinely live for 70 or 80 days, nearly twice the average Drosophila life span. Here evolutionary biologist Michael Rose has bred the long-lived stocks by selecting and mating flies late in life.

To begin the process of genetic selection, Rose first collected eggs laid by middle-aged fruit flies and let them hatch in isolation. The progeny were then transferred to a communal plexiglass cage to eat, grow, and breed under conditions ideal for mating. Once they had reached advanced ages, the eggs laid by older females (and fertilized by older males) were again collected and removed to individual hatching vials. The cycle was repeated, but with succeeding generations, the day on which the eggs were collected was progressively postponed. After two years and 15 generations, the laboratory had stocks of Drosophila with longer life spans.

The next question is what genes and what gene products are involved? Since the first experiments, Rose has bred longer life spans into fruit flies by selecting for other characteristics, such as ability to resist starvation, so the flies' long life spans are not necessarily tied to their fertility late in life.

One possibility is that the anti oxidant enzyme, superoxide dismutase (SOD), is involved. In another laboratory at Irvine the late Robert Tyler discovered that the longer-lived flies had a somewhat different form of the SOD gene, which was more active than its counterpart in the flies with average life spans. This finding has given a boost to the hypothesis that anti-oxidant enzymes like SOD are linked to aging or longevity.

Some of the genes found in yeast and fruit flies seem to promote longevity. But others may shorten life span. One such "death gene" has been isolated in nematodes by researchers at the University of

Colorado in Boulder, who found that mutation of a certain gene more than doubles the nematode's normal 3-week life span. Thomas Johnson's laboratory in Boulder has also uncovered evidence that the mutant may extend life span by overproducing superoxide dismutase (SOD) and catalase, two anti-oxidant enzymes that have been linked to longevity in other studies (see Oxygen Radicals).

The genes isolated so far are only a few of what scientists think may be dozens, perhaps hundreds, of longevity- and aging-related genes. Tracking them down in organisms like nematodes and yeast is just the beginning. The next big question for many gerontologists is whether there are counterparts in people — human homologs — of the genes found in laboratory animals.

Other unanswered questions concern the roles played by these genes. What exactly do they do? On one level, all genes function by transcribing their "codes" — actually DNA base sequences — into another nucleic acid called messenger ribonucleic acid or mRNA. Messenger RNA is then translated into proteins. Transcription and translation together constitute the process known as gene expression.

The proteins expressed by genes carry out a multitude of functions in each cell and tissue in the body, and some of these functions are related to aging. So when we ask what longevity- or aging-related genes do, we are actually asking what their protein products do at the cellular and tissue levels. Increasingly, gerontologists are also asking how alterations in the process of gene expression itself may affect aging.

Some proteins, such as anti oxidants, appear to prevent damage to cells, and others may repair damaged DNA or help cells respond to stress; more about these comes later. Other gene products are thought to control cell senescence, a process that could prove to be a key piece in the puzzle of aging and longevity.

Cell Senescence

Picture a cell: the threadlike pairs of chromosomes inhabit a nucleus that floats in a sea of cytoplasm along with other tiny organelles that do the cell's work, the whole cell is surrounded by and receives messages from other cells. Then picture the chromosomes, condensing into rod-like structures that divide in two, the nucleus disappearing, the chromosomes migrating to opposite sides of the cell where other nuclei are formed, and after that the entire cell following the chromosomes' lead, pulling apart and forming two identical daughter cells.

This, the process of mitosis, or asexual cell division, takes place in nearly all of the 100 trillion or so cells that make up the human body. But it does not go on indefinitely. About the middle of this century, researchers learned that cells have finite life spans, at least when studied in test tubes — in vitro. After a certain number of divisions, they enter a state of cell senescence, in which they do not divide or proliferate and DNA synthesis is blocked. For example, young human fibroblasts divide about 50 times and then stop. This phenomenon has become known as the Hayflick limit, after Leonard Hayflick, who with Paul Moorhead first described it while at the Wistar Institute in Philadelphia.

Intrigued by the possibility that the Hayflick limit might help explain some aspects of bodily aging, gerontologists have looked for and found links between senescence and human life spans. Fibroblasts taken from 75 year olds, for example, have fewer divisions remaining than cells from a child. Moreover, the longer a species' life span, the higher its Hayflick limit; human fibroblasts have higher Hayflick limits than mice fibroblasts.

Proliferative Genes

Searching for explanations of proliferation and senescence, scientists have found certain genes that appear to trigger cell proliferation. One example of such a short-lived protein is thought to regulate the expression of other genes important in cell division.

But c-fos and others of its kind are countered by anti-proliferative genes, which seem to interfere with division. The first evidence of an anti-proliferative gene came from an eye tumor called retinoblastoma. When one of the genes from retinoblastoma cells — later called the RB gene — became inactive, the cells went on dividing indefinitely and produced a tumor. But when the RB gene product was activated, the cells stopped dividing. This gene's product, in other words, appeared to suppress proliferation.

Senescence is the norm in the world of cells. In some cases, however, a cell somehow escapes this control mechanism and goes on dividing, becoming, in the terms of cell biology, immortal. And because immortal cells eventually form tumors, this is one area in which aging research and cancer research intersect. Investigators theorize that a failure of anti-proliferative genes (also known as tumor suppressor genes) is the first step in a complex process that leads to development of a tumor. Senescence, according to this view, may have evolved because it protected against cancer.

Still a mystery is how these genes' products function to promote and suppress cell proliferation. There are indications that a multilayer control system is at work, involving probably a host of intricate mechanisms that interact to maintain a balance between the two kinds of genes. Many gerontologists are now involved in unraveling these intricacies, studying both the genes and their products to learn which ones influence senescence and how.

Tracking Down a Longevity Gene

Investigators are finding clues to aging and longevity in yeast, one-celled organisms that have some intriguing genetic similarities to human cells. In a laboratory at Louisiana State University Medical Center in New Orleans, Micha Jazwinski has found genes that seem to promote longevity in these rapidly dividing, easy-to-study organisms.

Yeast normally have about 21 cell divisions or generations. Jazwinski observed that over the course of that "life span," certain genes in the yeast are more active or less active as the cells age; in the language of molecular biology, they are differentially expressed. So far, Jazwinski has found 14 such genes in yeast.

Selecting one of these genes, Jazwinski tried two different experiments. First, he introduced the gene into yeast cells in a form that allowed him to control its activity. When the gene was activated to a greater degree than normal, or overexpressed, some of the yeast cells went on dividing for 27 or 28 generations; their period of activity was extended by 30 percent. In his second experiment, Jazwinski mutated the gene. When he introduced this non-working version into a group of yeast cells, they had only about 12 divisions.

The two experiments made it clear that the gene, now called LAG-1, influences the number of divisions in yeast or, according to some researchers' ways of thinking, its longevity. (LAG-1 is short for longevity assurance gene.) But how it works is still a mystery. One small clue lies in its sequence of DNA bases — its genetic code — which suggests that it produces a protein found in cell membranes.

One next step is to study the function of that protein. Similar sequences have been found in human DNA, so a second investigative path is to clone the human gene and study its function. If there turns out to be a human LAG-1 counterpart, new insights into aging may be uncovered.

Telomeres

In the meantime, scientists are finding more clues to senescence in the architecture of DNA. Every chromosome, they have discovered, has tails at the ends that get shorter as a cell divides. Named telomeres, the tails all have the same, short sequence of DNA bases repeated thousands of times. The repetitive structure stabilizes the chromosomes, forming a tight bond between the two strands of the DNA.

Each time a cell divides, the telomeres shed a number of bases, so telomere length gives some indication of how many divisions the cell has already undergone and how many remain before it becomes senescent. This apparent counting mechanism, almost like an abacus keeping track of the cell's age, has led to speculation that telomeres do serve as molecular meters of cell division. But they may play a more active role, and telomere researchers are exploring the possibility that these chromosome ends regulate cellular life span in some way.

Telomere research is another territory where cancer and aging research merge. In immortal cancer cells, telomeres act abnormally — they stop shrinking with each cell division. In the search for clues to this phenomenon, researchers have zeroed in on an enzyme called telomerase.

Normally absent in adult cells, telomerase seems to swing into action in advanced cancers, enabling the telomeres to replace lost sequences and divide indefinitely. This finding has led to speculation that if a drug could be developed to block telomerase activity, it might aid in cancer treatment. Whether cell senescence is explained by abnormal gene products, telomere shortening, or other factors, the question of what senescence has to do with the aging of organisms remains and continues to be the focus of intense study.

In the meantime, gerontologists are also studying proteins in the body that may play a role in aging and longevity. Genes hold the codes to these proteins, but what substances turn the genes on and off? And once activated, how do their products interact with the products of other genes? What is their effect on cells and tissues? The biochemistry of aging holds some of the answers.

Growing Replacement Organs

In an amazing leap forward in medical and biological technology, scientists have developed the ability to grow replacement organs for animals, using cells taken from those animals. Scientists have successfully grown organs for sheep, rats and rabbits. They place cells taken from the animals into molds which take the shape of hearts, kidneys and bladders.

Scientists have also found ways to grow new skin and bone cartilage from just a few cells taken from full grown animals. The goal is to create a steady supply of "off-the-shelf" body parts which can be used to replace sick and diseased organs in people, without the need for a donor organ from another person. Medical researchers have already successfully grown and replaced a bladder and a windpipe is a sheep, a kidney for a rat and leg muscles for a rabbit. The tissue to grow the organs was taken from newborn animals and fetuses.

The researchers have also developed a method for replacing organs in fetuses before they are born, opening the door for a dramatic new technology in the prevention of birth defects. Doctors eventually want to be able to examine a fetus, discover problems, and fix the problem long before the baby enters the world.

For example, if an examination discovers that a fetus has a faulty heart, doctors would remove a few cells from the heart, place them in a mold in a laboratory setting, and grow a new healthy heart. The new heart would be transplanted into the growing fetus, which would then complete its development in the womb, and ideally, be born in a state of perfect health.

While researchers have already successfully completed this amazing feat in animals, they are seeking to begin the first organ growth and replacement in human beings. Researchers at Cornell University say growing new organs from the original body is a way to solve one of the biggest drawbacks to current organ transplant operations — rejection of the foreign organ or tissue by the host.

Conducting surgery on tiny, developing fetuses is extremely tricky work. It requires the use of microscopes and tiny surgical instruments which are extremely difficult to manipulate by the hands of a surgeon. Doctors use ultrasound to detect birth defects as early as three months into pregnancy. If defects are found, they wait until the baby is six months along. Then, through small incisions, they insert a surgical camera and long, narrow instruments into the womb. Guided by a computer video monitor, they remove a pea-sized sample of the tissue from the organ in question. The mother is given drugs to prevent labor.

With the tissue samples in hand, surgeons separate out different cells from the tissue sample and place the ones they want into a glass dish filled with a solution of proteins and other nutrients needed to keep the cells alive and multiplying. The organ then grows at a rate much more rapid than the normal development of the organ. Before long, it's time to re-enter the womb and replace the organ of the soon-to-be newborn baby. **If everything goes right, the baby will be born in a state of 100 percent health.**

The implications of this technology are wide-ranging and astounding. If researchers develop the ability to grow new organs for fetuses, it is a short leap to growing new organs for adults using a similar process.

Many believe we are on the threshold of developing the ability to grow just about any body part or tissue to replace the diseased or worn out part of any human being. Imagine replacing the pancreas of a diabetic, curing that person of his disease by providing him with a proper insulin producing organ that keeps his blood sugars in balance. Imagine an 80-year-old man dying from lung cancer, and replacing those diseased and damaged lungs with fresh, new, healthy lungs — grown from cells that were taken from his own body. That means there needs to be no outside donor, no fear of rejection — just a new chance at life where previously only a certain death could be expected.

Organ replacement technology is another piece in the puzzle of finding a true Fountain of Youth. This technology may enable human being to shatter the 120-130 maximum life span barrier, with a maximum lifespan extending to truly amazing possibilities of longevity.

Chapter 10

The Secrets of a Youthful Brain

C hildren are amazing. Their energy is endless. Their minds are crisp, sharp, clear and so curious it almost hurts. **A youthful mind is a true wonder — a thing of beauty.** For many people of advanced age, it seems difficult to believe that they at one time had the very same kind of mental ability. You were able to remember names, dates, phone numbers, even the address of your second cousin in Dayton.

With age, many people find that what they once took for granted — a sharp mind — has somehow slowly slipped away from them. With each passing year, you use more and more little crutches for your mind. A notebook to help you remember names and important dates. Leaving Post-It notes all over the house to make sure you don't forget important meetings and tasks you want to get done that day. Or tying the proverbial string around the finger.

In addition to a slipping memory, many elderly people find it more difficult to solve complex problems, to think clearly about things which other people take for granted, and to maintain focused concentration for long periods of time. Like a muscle that has gone flabby and which can no longer lift a heavy weight, the mental muscle seems to have lost its ability to do "heavy thinking."

More and more, you are asking your kids to help balance your checkbook. You are asking for advice on how to cope with everyday mental tasks, such as reading and understanding your life insurance policy, figuring your income tax return or understanding what your doctor is telling you.

The Brain

Before we talk about how to maintain a youthful mind and brain, a little brain primer is in order. It will help you understand how to keep you brain young, and why what we are going to suggest works.

Basically, the brain is made up of three distinct part which are connected. They are the cerebrum, the cerebellum, and the brain stem.

Also called the medulla oblongata, the term brain stem usually refers to all the structures lying between the cerebrum and the spinal cord, that is, the diencephalon, midbrain, pons, and medulla. These parts all arise from the embryonic forebrain, midbrain, or hindbrain. In addition, although the brain is well protected by the cranium, it is covered by three membranes called meninges. The outer one, the dura mater, is tough and shiny. The middle membrane, the arachnoid layer, encloses the brain loosely and does not slip down into the brain's convolutions, or ridges. The inner membrane, the pia mater, consists mainly of small blood vessels that adhere to the surface of the brain.

The Key to the Thinking Process: Neurons

It's an unfortunate fact of life that the brain shrinks as we grow older. The key element in this shrinking process is the neuron. A neuron is a long cell that has a thick central area containing the nucleus; it also has one long process called an axon and one or more short, bushy processes called dendrites.

Dendrites receive impulses from other neurons. These impulses are sent electrically along the cell membrane to the end of the axon. At the tip of the axon the signal is chemically transmitted to an adjacent neuron or muscle cell.

Neurons have a negative electrical charge inside the cell membrane. Scientists call this polarization. This is due to the free movement of positively charged potassium ions through the cell membrane and, at the same time, the retention of large, negatively charged molecules within the cell. Positively charged sodium ions are kept outside the cell by an active process.

All cells have this charge difference, but when a stimulating current is applied to a nerve cell, a unique event occurs. First, potassium ions flow into the cell, reducing the negative charge. At a certain point the properties of the membrane change and the cell becomes permeable to sodium, which rapidly enters the cell and causes a net positive charge inside the neuron. This is called the action potential.

Once this potential is reached at one area in the neuron, it travels down the axon by ion exchange at specific points, called nodes of Ranvier. The size of the action potential is self-limiting, because a high internal sodium concentration causes the pumping out first of potassium and then of sodium ions, restoring the negative charge inside the cell membrane, that is the neuron is repolarized. The whole process takes less than one-thousandth of a second. After a very brief period, called the refractory period, the neuron can repeat this process.

Two types of phenomena are involved in processing brain activity: electrical and chemical. Electrical events create a signal within a neuron, and chemical processes transmit the signal from one neuron to another neuron or to a muscle cell.

When the electrical signal reaches the tip of an axon, it stimulates small presynaptic vesicles in the cell. These vesicles contain chemicals called neurotransmitters, which are released into the submicroscopic space between neurons. The neurotransmitters attach to specialized receptors on the surface of the adjacent neuron. This stimulus causes the adjacent cell to depolarize and propagate an action potential of its own. The duration of a stimulus from a neurotransmitter is limited by the breakdown of the chemicals in the synaptic cleft and the reuptake by the neuron that produced them. Formerly, each neuron was thought to make only one transmitter, but recent studies have shown that some cells make two or more.

The Brain Shrinks

By age 70, the average person has lost some one billion neurons. Fortunately, the brain has some 10 billion neurons, so even a loss of 10 percent does not mean a total debilitation of the functioning of the brain. Yet, if you had your choice, you certainly would not choose to lose 10 percent of the functioning of your very own brain — the seat of your soul, your mind, your personhood, all your feelings, all your memories, everything that makes you the person you truly are.

Those people who live beyond age 70 start to experience an even greater loss of neurons. Those who live to age 90 lose a whopping 4 billion neurons, or some 40 percent of the brain's total supply of these vital cells. It's a small wonder that so many people who reach a very old age are so often completely senile. They can't remember their own name, no longer recognize their own children or other loved ones, have no idea where they are or who they are.

Still, not all people who live to a very old age "go senile," yet they still have lost a large percentage of their neuron supply.

Why do some people maintain the use of their mind with such a diminished capacity of neuron supply?

As it happens, Mother Nature has a plan to make up for the steady loss of neurons in the brain. When a neuron dies, the others around it actually expand and take over part of the functioning of the lost cell. Medical doctors call this reactive synaptogenesis, which is a fancy way of saying that as some cells die, others expand and spread out to take over for the lost soldier.

Many doctors now believe that the No. 1 cause of senile dementia, Alzheimer's Disease, may in fact be a more rapid acceleration of the aging process in which neurons die off on cue as the years roll by.

Now the good news. We no longer have to sit by and let our brain cells die as we age. In fact, rather than losing brain cells as we grow older, we cannot only stop the process of neural die-off in its tracks, we can actually build more complex connections between the neurons, making the brain even more complete and powerful as we advance into our 90s, and 100s! Yes, it's true!

Growing old and losing one's mind simply does not have to be!! Let us repeat: Just because you are getting on in years, does not mean that you cannot have the springy mental capability of any 19 year old. It's an absolute fact. Old age DOES NOT equal weak mind.

Anyone who does not have an actual disease or damage to the brain should maintain a crisp, healthy alert mind for as long as they live, even if they live to be 120 or older. Need we remind you that the world's oldest woman, Jeanne Calment of France recorded a rap music CD at age 121!! She not only performed every song on the CD, she also wrote and produced them. Not bad for 121!

So how do we do it? What measures can we take to not only stop the brain from deteriorating, but to make it actually grow stronger as we age? The first answer lies in nutrition, or more exactly, feeding the brain the nutrients it needs so that its billions of neurons can go right on functioning for more than a century.

Fortunately, modern science, ancient medicine and Mother Nature have joined forces to provide us with a substance that is so powerful, it may be the only one thing we need to keep the brain in tip top condition for as long as the human body continues to function. **What is this amazing substance? It's Ginkgo Biloba.**

The Ultimate Brain Rejuvenator

For literally thousands of years, ancient healers have known about a certain tree which contains a substance that has at least a dozen different healing and restorative effects on the human body, especially the mind and brain.

The ginkgo tree is an amazing entity in its own right. This unbelievably hardy tree has survived at least one quarter of a billion years on this planet, living through droughts and ice ages, catastrophic extinction of millions of other species and a variety of other earth-shattering events, including asteroid strikes, comet collisions and massive cosmic radiation bursts from outer space.

In fact, the ginkgo tree is so tough and hardy, it was the only living thing to survive the atomic blasts and annihilations of the two Japanese cities — Hiroshima and Nagasaki — during World War II. At Hiroshima, observers noted that a single ginkgo tree was the only living thing at ground zero, the very spot below which the atomic bomb exploded.

Furthermore, scientists have identified individual ginkgo trees that are more than 1,000 years old! These trees are not only incredibly resistant to adverse environmental conditions, they have the ability to live on and on, century after century.

Ginkgos are planted as hardy shade trees in many places in the world, especially in cities, partly because they are so resistant to insects, bacteria, viruses, pollution and even old age.

Now, scientists believe that people who eat the products of these trees — including its nuts and leaves — will absorb much of its incredible strength and power of longevity.

For thousands of years, the people of China, who have always recognized the tree's unique stamina and longevity, have used ginkgo nuts for thousands of years as a remedy for cancer, venereal disease, asthma, lung weakness and congestion, impaired hearing and to increase sexual energy and generally promote longevity.

Today the ancient ginkgo has sparked renewed interest throughout the world because medical researchers have isolated chemical compounds from ginkgo that show startling effects in humans. These compounds regulate blood flow to the brain, legs and other extremities and control levels of various neurotransmitters in the brain, thus helping to counteract memory loss, depression and lack of alertness which may develop in old age. These same compounds also block a substance called platelet activating factor (PAF) which, by over-stimulating the immune system, may lead to conditions such as asthma, toxic shock from bacterial poisons and perhaps even atherosclerosis and stroke.

Here is a quick outlines of what ginkgo biloba can do for the human body:

● Improves the condition of the blood. Thins the blood viscosity and lowers platelet adhesiveness; protects red blood cells by stabilizing their membranes; increases blood vessel tone; stabilizes capillary permeability.

● Free-radical scavenger. Protects cell membranes in the brain and other tissues throughout the body against free-radical damage. Cell membranes are particularly sensitive to free-radical damage, which can lead to destruction of the entire cell.

● Increases the uptake and utilization of oxygen and glucose in tissues throughout the body.

● Increases blood flow to the brain and extremities.

● Regulates or increases brain metabolism. This counteracts depression and is one of a variety of other mental disorders which result from sluggish brain metabolism.

● Regulates neurotransmitters. Neurotransmitters are chemicals which carry the very thought of the brain. Interrupted flow of these vital brain chemicals can lead to problems at the most fundamental level of human thought. People with disrupted neurotransmitter flow may not feel like themselves, be depressed, suffer memory loss or become senile.

● Protects myelin. Myelin is the protective coating which covers the nerves, protecting them from outside damage and encasing them in such a way that makes for efficient flow of electrical impulses throughout the body. Diseases such as muscular dystrophy occur when, for some reason, the myelin begins to deteriorate, disrupting nerve transmission to the muscles, making them weak and ultimately useless. Ginkgo may be an effective agent in helping people with MD regain some of their lost mobility, or prevent further loss of muscle use.

● Protects hearing. Helps protect against and even restore impaired hearing, especially when due to damage from loud noise or infection.

● Shows anti-bacterial and anti-candida activity.

Under modern laboratory study, ginkgo has been found to be an effective remedy for general lack of alertness, not only in elderly people, but in other people who seem slow of thought and mind.

Ginkgo is also effective against a variety of allergies and against asthma. Because it increases the flow of blood to the brain, it helps people with Alzheimer's Disease regain some of the lost cognition they have suffered due to the massive loss of neurons in their brains.

Ginkgo has been shown to help people recover from problems with dizziness, or vertigo, usually caused by imbalances of the fluids in the ears. For some reason, ginkgo helps restore inner-ear fluid to their proper level of balance. Ginkgo has also been shown to restore hearing loss in some individuals, which again may have something to do with the fluids of the inner ears. Ear ringing, also known as tinnitus, is another problem ginkgo seems able to clear up.

So ginkgo is effective against ringing in the ears (tinnitus), disturbance of balance, dizziness (vertigo), sudden hearing loss and hearing weakness. All may all result from lack of proper blood circulation. These conditions can also be caused by free radical damage.

Ginkgo is an extremely effective agent for producing more efficient blood flow through the entire body. It helps blood flow more freely by making it less sticky, which can prevent heart disease and strokes, and also delivers more oxygen to every cell in the human body, making them more efficient and energetic.

Increased blood flow the brain also means easing of depression for many people who suffer from this very common disorder which afflicts 47 million Americans on any given day. Decreased blood flow to the brain can adversely affect memory, concentration, intellectual ability, vision, equilibrium and balance. It may also lead to symptoms such as headaches, depression and mental confusion. Stroke can occur because of lack of blood flow and oxygen to brain tissue. Ginkgo is used to prevent and even treat all of these conditions.

Because many sexual problems in men are caused by disruptions in blood flow to the penis, ginkgo, which helps stimulate blood flow throughout the entire body, can be a very effective treatment for sexual impotence.

In China, people eat ginkgo nuts for their good taste and for their strengthening and tonic properties. Ginkgo nuts are used as a kidney yang tonic, which means that they are capable of increasing sexual energy, stopping bed-wetting, restoring hearing loss and soothing bladder irritation. When boiled as a tea, the nuts are also thought to be a good remedy for lung weakness and congestion — particularly coughs and asthma. When used on a regular basis, they can also help control vaginal candidiasis ("yeast infection"), frequent urination, cloudy urine and excess mucous in the urinary tract. Other common uses for ginkgo include eating the cooked nuts as a remedy for intestinal worms, cancer, gonorrhea and leukorrhea, and using them as a poultice for infections (modern studies have demonstrated antibiotic activity).

Ginkgo leaves are used for treating chilblains (reddening, swelling and itching of the skin due to frostbite), while a tea of the leaves is sprayed into the throat for asthma. Modern laboratory studies with humans have found compounds in ginkgo leaves called ginkgolides can reduce the bronchial reactivity of asthmatic patients to common allergens such as dust and pollen. Other compounds (called terpenes) have the ability to block the production of platelet activating factor (PAF), one of the primary agents responsible for bronchial reactivity.

Proper blood circulation is essential for good health and cannot be overemphasized how vital it is to our health and well-being. How freely blood can move through the vessels to all parts of the body and how well it can carry nutrients (such as oxygen, sugars, enzymes and other life-giving nutrients) and remove the waste products of cellular metabolism directly affects the health of every cell in the body.

When these nutrients, oxygen, sugars and enzymes are not supplied to the cells of the body continuously throughout the day and night, and the wastes are not constantly removed, something very dramatic happens: All the cells of the body begin to age more rapidly. For when our cells, tissues and organs are not properly nourished and sit in their own wastes, they wear out much faster. We begin to experience aches and pains, we get stiff, our joints start to weaken, and we have trouble running and walking. Stress, poor diet, injury and lack of exercise can all cause our circulation to diminish.

When our brain also starts to become less alive, it forgets the name of our childhood friend, forgets and doesn't learn new things as well, and has trouble keeping up with all the changes going on around us. We say, "We are starting to get old."

In Europe herbal medicine is more developed and accepted by both the public and health care professionals than in the US. Extracts made from ginkgo leaves are among the best-selling herbal medicinal products. Laboratory studies have found that an extract of ginkgo improves brain functioning in the young and old, prevents or treats circulatory disorders such as stroke and arterial insufficiency (lack of adequate blood supply to the extremities) and can be of use in treating and protecting against hearing disorders, macular degeneration in the eye, and possibly asthma.

Ginkgo may be the ideal herbal support to counteract some of the most common conditions associated with the aging process and with environmental pollution and stress. With regular use, Ginkgo can help increase and maintain the blood supply to all the tissues of the body, but especially to the brain, extremities, skin, eyes, inner ear, heart and other vital organs.

Ginkgo is a powerful weapon for people who suffer from circulation disorders. Peripheral vascular disease may cause poor circulation in the legs, making walking difficult. It may also cause poor circulation to the skin, heart and other organs.

Finally, ginkgo may be a new and powerful weapon in certain disorders of the eye. The retina may be damaged by free radicals, hemorrhage (as in senile macular degeneration) and perhaps restricted circulation due to stress. Ginkgo reverses the conditions which lead to all these problems, primarily by scrubbing the body of free radicals and improving blood flow in the tiny capillaries that supply the eyes with blood.

To sum up:

Ginkgo has three main effects on the body:

1) Improves and enhances circulation to all cells and to all the vital tissues and organs of the body, especially the heart and the brain, which result in overall greater health, clearer thinking and more energy.

2) Scrubs free radicals from the body. Free radicals are molecules which break down cell structure at an extreme, or atomic level, which most medical researchers now believe is the central element of the aging process. Fewer free radicals means slower aging. Ginkgo does that for you.

3) Ginkgo blocks a substance in our body called platelet-activating factor, also known as PAF, which many doctors believe contributes to such problems as asthma, heart disease, hearing disorders and skin disorders, including psoriasis.

And the bottom line is ...

Ginkgo will preserve your brain and help keep your mind young. It will prevent loss of neurons. Instead of losing 1 to 4 billion of your 10 billion neurons, you may lose zero, and even gain existing neuron branches, making your brain more powerful as you grow older.

Other Dietary Factors for a Young Brain

Now that you know about the virtual miracle of ginkgo biloba, it will be helpful to look at many other factors which can help the brain grow old and deteriorate — or stay young and healthy for years to come.

For example, all the evidence seems to suggest that a high fat diet is conducive to poor brain functioning. In other words, the more fatty meats and sweets you eat, the greater the chance your brain is going to take an early slow down in your life. Switching to a low-fat diet may add years to the healthy functioning of your brain.

Your brain will also benefit greatly from healthy doses of substances that are known as antioxidants. We have talked about these substances a lot throughout this book, and they make their appearance again for good reason here as we talk about a young, healthy brain. The brain contains a lot of cells which contain fat, which is especially susceptible to free-radical damage, and thus, brain deterioration.

So make sure you take your daily doses of foods that are high in the major antioxidants — vitamin C, E, A and beta carotene. Also trace elements, especially zinc and selenium, are excellent preservers of brain structure and functioning.

In fact, trace elements are other inorganic substances that appear in the body in minute amounts and are essential for health of the brain. Little is known about how they function in the brain, and most knowledge about them comes from how their absence, especially in animals, affects health. Trace elements appear in sufficient amounts in most foods. But one thing is clear — the brain would not be able to function without trace elements

Among the more important trace elements for brain functioning and brain health is copper, which is present in many enzymes and in copper-containing proteins found in the blood, brain, and liver. Copper deficiency is associated with the failure to use iron in the formation of hemoglobin. Zinc is also important in forming enzymes. Deficiency in zinc is believed to impair growth and, in severe cases, to cause dwarfism.

Fluorine, which is retained especially in the teeth and bones, has been found necessary for growth in animals. Fluorides, a category of fluorine compounds, are important for protecting against demineralization of bone. The fluoridation of water supplies has proved an effective measure against tooth decay, reducing it by as much as 40 percent. Other trace elements include chromium, molybdenum, and selenium.

All of the above must be present in sufficient amounts to maintain a lasting and healthy brain that functions as it should.

By the way, zinc is especially important and is a substance the brain absolutely must have to grow and maintain healthy functioning. That's because this rare metal in the human body plays a vital role in the flow of neurotransmmittres, the most important chemicals of the human brain.

Zinc deficiency is known to cause depression and other kinds of mental illness, even some severe mental illnesses, such as bipolar disorders, amnesia, hallucinations and more. One of the primary ways in which the human body loses zinc is through stress. A hectic lifestyle results in the production of stress chemicals in the body, one of which is called cryptopyyrole. This substance attaches itself to zinc molecules, along with vitamin B6, and causes them to be expelled out of the system.

Another important brain element is lecithin, a substance which contains something called choline. In tests on both animals and humans, choline has been shown to improve memory, produce higher scores on mental skills tests and provide for overall maximized brain production. Lecithin also increases another vital neurotransmitter called acetycholine. **Another vitally important brain booster is an amino acid called tryptophan.**

First, what is an amino acid?

Amino acids are a fundamental important class of organic compounds that contain both the amino and carboxyl groups. There more than 150 different kinds of amino acids, but 20 of them make up one of the building blocks of the brain and body — good old protein. These are called standard or alphaamino acids. They are: **alanine, arginine, asparagine, aspartic acid, cysteine, glutamic acid, glutamine, glycine, histidine, isoleucine, leucine, lysine, methionine, phenylalanine, proline, serine, threonine, tryptophan, tyrosine, and valine.**

When a living cell makes protein, the carboxyl group of one amino acid is linked to the amino group of another to form what is called a peptide bond. The carboxyl group of the second amino acid is similarly linked to the amino group of a third, and so on, until a long chain is produced. This chainlike molecule, which may contain from 50 to several hundred amino acid subunits, is called a polypeptide.

A protein may be formed of a single polypeptide chain, or it may consist of several such chains held together by weak molecular bonds. Each protein is formed according to a precise set of instructions contained within the nucleic acid, which is the genetic material of the cell.

These instructions determine which of the 20 standard amino acids are to be incorporated into the protein, and in what sequence. The R groups of the amino acid subunits determine the final shape of the protein and its chemical properties; an extraordinary variety of proteins can be produced from the same 20 subunits. The standard amino acids serve as raw materials for the manufacture of many other cellular products, including hormones and pigments. In addition, several of these amino acids are key intermediates in cellular metabolism.

Most plants and microorganisms are able to use inorganic compounds to make all the amino acids they require for normal growth. Animals, however, must obtain some of the standard amino acids from their diet in order to survive; these particular amino acids are called essential. Essential amino acids for humans include lysine, tryptophan, valine, histidine, leucine, isoleucine, phenylalanine, threonine, methionine, and arginine. They are found in adequate amounts in protein-rich foods from animal sources or in carefully chosen combinations of plant proteins.

One amino acid listed above, tryptophan, helps the brain produce serotonin, which is an extremely important neurotransmitter which helps regulate sleep, mental stability, pain levels and anxiety. People with inadequate serotonin levels may be easily subject to inexplicable panic and anxiety attacks.

Brain serotonin is necessary for normal sleep to occur, although it is only one of many elements and is not sufficient in itself. The roles that two other chemicals, norepinephrine and dopamine, have in sleep are less certain. Several brain chemicals called biogenic amines — dopamine, norepinephrine, and serotonin — act as neurotransmitters and neuro-modulators in regulating discharge of brain cells. But the evidence is best that serotonin is the true key in this process, and thus, you need this vital element to have a healthy brain and mind.

Iodine

Iodine is a critical brain nutrient. People who are deficient of iodine can develop a condition called cretinism, a major attribute of which is impaired brain functioning.

Cretins have dwarfed bodies, with curvature of the spine and pendulous abdomen. Their limbs are distorted, their features are coarse, and their hair is harsh and scanty. Mental development is retarded throughout life. An adult cretin may reach the intelligence of only a four-year-old child. Research has revealed that when an animal or human infant is born with a deficiency of thyroxine, the neurons (nerve cells) in the brain do not develop the multiple branches that normally form the brain's complex network.

B Is for Brain

Those class of vitamins known as the B vitamins — B1, B2, B3, B5, B6, B12, and folacin, or folic acid — might as well stand for brain vitamins because they are so entirely essential for a healthy brain that will stay young for many years.

Collectively, these are generally called B complex. They are particularly important to carbohydrate metabolism, the process which turns food into energy which the brain and the rest of the body can use.

B1

B1 is more commonly called thiamine, and it is a colorless, crystalline substance, acts as a catalyst in carbohydrate metabolism, and also plays a role in the synthesis of nerve-regulating substances. A brain deficient in thiamin is weak and unable to process energy properly enough to allow for normal every day thinking to go on without a hitch.

Brain food rich in thiamine are pork, organ meats (liver, heart, and kidney), brewer's yeast, lean meats, eggs, leafy green vegetables, whole or enriched cereals, wheat germ, berries, nuts, and legumes.

By the way, the reason why white flour and that which is made from it — breads, sweet rolls, pancakes — are bad for the body and the brain is the fact that thiamine has been removed from it in the milling process. **Thus, if you want to feed your brain properly, avoid white flour and sweet rolls in favor of thiamine rich whole wheat bread, brown rice and other products made only from whole grain.**

B2

B2 is more commonly called riboflavin and works closely with thiamine to help keep the brain supplied with and processing energy. The best food sources of riboflavin are liver, milk, meat, dark green vegetables, whole grain and enriched cereals, pasta, bread, and mushrooms.

B3

B3 is more commonly called niacin and works as a coenzyme in the brain to release the energy of nutrients which are transported to the brain by the blood. A deficiency of niacin causes mental confusion, irritability, and, when the central nervous system is affected, depression and mental disturbances.

The best food sources of niacin are liver, poultry, meat, canned tuna and salmon, whole grain and enriched cereals, dried beans and peas, and nuts. The body also makes niacin from the amino acid tryptophan, the very important amino acid which which we talked about above. Large doses of niacin have been used to treat such devastating brain diseases as schizophrenia, although the effectiveness of this treatment is still under investigation. Be careful with megadosing this substance, however, because it can causes liver damage if taken in large doses over long periods of time.

B6

Vitamin B6 is necessary for the absorption and metabolism of amino acids, which we have already discussed, are essential for building the proteins which make up the very substance of the brain. A deficiency of B6 is characterized by convulsions, dizziness, nausea, anemia, and kidney stones. The best food sources of B6 are whole grains, cereals, bread, liver, avocados, spinach, green beans, and bananas. **All excellent brain foods.**

B12

B12 is necessary in tiny amounts for the formation of nucleoproteins, proteins, and red blood cells, and for the functioning of the nervous system — the core operating system of a healthy brain.

Food which contain liberal amounts of B12 are liver, kidneys, meat, fish, eggs, and milk. Note: People who maintain a vegetarian diet would be well advised to take B12 supplements to maintain a healthy brain over a long period of time.

Folic acid is a coenzyme needed for forming body protein and hemoglobin. Dietary sources are organ meats, leafy green vegetables, legumes, nuts, whole grains, and brewer's yeast. Folic acid is lost in foods stored at room temperature and during cooking.

Pantothenic acid, another B vitamin, plays a still-undefined role in the metabolism of proteins, carbohydrates, and fats. It is abundant in many foods and is manufactured by intestinal bacteria as well.

The Bad Metals

We told you about the heavy metals that the brain must have to function at peak performance levels — zinc, copper, manganese and iron.

But there are other metals which are just the opposite of being brain friendly — they can cause brain damage, insanity, mental retardation, or simply poor and fuzzy thinking.

The real bad heavy metals of the brain are: aluminum, mercury, lead and cadmium.

Lead poisoning is a well-known cause of both mental retardation and insanity. In fact, some historians have suggested that the infamous and insane Roman emperor, Nero, the man who played the fiddle while Rome burned, may have lost his mind because he drank his wine from a goblet made of lead. Trace portions of the lead were dissolved by the alcohol in the wine, which allowed the metal to get into Emperor Nero's brain wiring, making him irrational and psychotic.

Today, public health officials are well aware of the damaging effects of lead on the brains of children. Many children who live in ghettos and old, inner-city buildings are exposed to old paint, which contains small amounts of lead. Just having casual contact with old paint dust can result in major brain damage in children, a condition from which they will suffer for the rest of their lives.

Another source of lead in the environment is gasoline, although most leaded gasoline has now been phased out of general use. Still, many decades of use of leaded gasoline has caused a lot of lead to be deposited and concentrated in some areas, such as the soil adjacent to heavily traveled roads and high-ways.

If you live near a heavily traveled road, and you have occasion to walk on the side of this road every day, you may be dragging lead into your house on the bottom of your shoes. This shoe-born lead can collect in greater and greater amounts on carpeting inside the house. Children, who frequently crawl or play on the carpet, can then ingest lead by putting their hands in their mouths — and potentially suffer damage to the brain.

Thus, it pays to make sure that your environment is free of lead, meaning you should never live in an apartment or house containing old paint or live near heavily traveled roads. Another area of high lead content is near airports. Some glazed pots and ceramic dishes can also contain trace amounts of lead, and a trace is all it takes to cause considerable damage to the brain.

Aluminum finds its way into the body in many ways. A lot of people believe that using aluminum pots and pans is a bad idea because tiny amounts of lead may move from the pan to your food and even-tually inside your system. Others dispute this, how-ever, and most experts believe that aluminum pots and pans are as safe as any.

Another possible source of aluminum are soda cans. Many people believe that drinking large amounts of acidic soft drinks can result in trace amounts of aluminum getting into the body and eventually the brain. Again, this is controversial, but some think it is a wise idea to avoid soft drinks for this very reason.

Many antiperspirants contain aluminum, and thus, many people avoid using them. Aluminum can be absorbed through the skin. Another common substance which contains aluminum are antacid tablets. Look on the label of antacids you consider buying. If they contain aluminum, you may want to avoid them to protect your brain.

Another possible and controversial source of heavy metal in the body are the very fillings in your teeth, which among other metals, contain silver. Silver, like lead and aluminum, is a poison to the brain. Modern dentists are using different alloys for fillings which do not contain silver, so you may want to consider having your old fillings removed and updated with materials that have no chance of causing problems. Of course, many dentists contend that there is no real proof that silver fillings cause any problems at all. More research still needs to be done to find answers.

What if you already have some of these metals in your body? Is there a way to detoxify? Yes, there are several things you can do to shed unwanted heavy metals from your system. First, go to your health food store and buy something called glutathione. This substance can scrub heavy metals from the brain. Another such substance is cysteine. Both of the above are amino acids which bind to heavy met-

als and flush them from your body. Good old vitamin C and selenium, the latter of which you can best
get by eating Brazil nuts, are also cleansers of heavy
metals from your brain.

**Speaking of vitamin C, this substance is extreme-
ly important in the maintenance of a healthy brain.**

Also known as ascorbic acid, this superstar of the
vitamins is important in the formation and maintenance of collagen, the protein that supports many
body structures, including elements of the brain.

It also enhances the absorption of iron from foods
of vegetable origin. Scurvy is the classic manifestation of severe ascorbic acid deficiency.

In some experiments ascorbic acid has been
shown to prevent the formation of nitrosamines
compounds found to produce tumors in laboratory
animals and possibly also in humans. Although
unused ascorbic acid is quickly excreted in the
urine, large and prolonged doses can result in the
formation of bladder and kidney stones, interference
with the effects of blood-thinning drugs, destruction
of B12, and the loss of calcium from bones.

Sources of vitamin C include citrus fruits, fresh
strawberries, cantaloupe, pineapple, and guava.
Good vegetable sources are broccoli, Brussels
sprouts, tomatoes, spinach, kale, green peppers,
cabbage, and turnips.

Vitamin C has a lot of enemies — they are copper,
alcohol, caffeine, aspirin, antibiotics and daily stress.

Because vitamin C cannot be manufactured by the human body, once a person burns what it has taken in, no more is available.

A body without vitamin C, even for an hour a day, is a body laid open to all kinds of problems, including deterioration of the brain.

Vitamin C deficiency is a well known cause of mental health problems which include mental fatigue, depression, dizziness, insomnia and Parkinson's disease, a brain disorder that causes severe convulsions and loss of coordination. Significantly, many patients diagnosed with schizophrenia are found to be chronically deficient of vitamin C.

In one fascinating experiment, schizophrenic patients were given massive doses of vitamin C, and all of them showed at least some improvement, with some showing significant improvement. Additionally, many anti-psychotic drugs are helped along and made more effective by vitamin C.

The great thing about vitamin C is that it is absorbed by your body like a food — meaning that it is almost impossible to overdose on this vitamin. Taking megadoses of vitamin C is generally considered to be safe, while taking large amounts of other vitamins can have toxic side effects, some of them quite severe.

Thus, take all the vitamin C you can each and every day — your brain will stay young and healthy as a result.

The Youthful Brain — Part II

Proper nutrition is not the only way in which we can keep the brain young and healthy for life.

The research is absolutely conclusive that an active, heavily used brain is also a brain that will stay sharp and healthy for as long as the human body lives. You must constantly challenge your brain by using it to think — but not just think — you must also challenge yourself with difficult mental problems to work on and solve.

If you think about it, this is just common sense! Like a muscle, the brain stays fit with use. If you don't exercise the muscles of your body on a regular basis, most of you will lose muscle mass, gain wait, get soft and flabby. In short, unused muscles respond by going flabby. Muscles that are used respond by getting thicker and harder.

This analogy is a direct correlation to the way the brain works. A brain that is underused is a brain that simply will not demonstrate peak performance. On the other hand, a brain that is constantly being challenged with tough problems is a brain that will be faster, smarter and more capable of solving problems, making quick decisions, remembering things with ease and engaging in creative production of anything from art to business dealings.

Recent studies with school children have concluded that playing chess, for example, results in better student performance on everyday school work. Students who were taught to play chess, and who were asked to play a specific amount of chess matches per week, saw their grade point average increase by a whopping 24 percent over students who did not play regular games of chess.

The reason the chess matches made the children smarter has to do with the kind of mental tasks the game of chess demands of the brain — thinking, strategizing, remembering, planning ahead, visualizing positions, inventing new plans of attack, and so on. While the actual goal of a game of chess — beating your opponent — has little to do with solving an algebra problem, the fact that the same kind of thinking processes must be used makes doing algebra easier.

Similarly, while lifting weights has little to do with playing the game of baseball, an athlete who lifts weights will most likely be a better overall player than those who do not lift weights because they will have stronger, better coordinated muscles, which can be used to perform any kind of athletic activity more efficiently.

Improving the Memory

The same goes for memory. A memory that is not used is a memory that goes soft. Very often, the reason elderly people experience failing memory is not because their brain is aging, but simply because they have retired from their jobs, and they no longer use their memories as rigorously as they did when doing so was often a make-it or break-it situation.

Before we talk about ways we can improve the memory of just about any human being, no matter how old they are, let's take a closer look to see what memory actually is, and how it works in the human brain.

Memory is the process of storing and retrieving information in the brain. The process is central to learning and thinking. Four different types of remembering are ordinarily distinguished by psychologists: recollection, recall, recognition, and relearning. Recollection involves the reconstruction of events or facts on the basis of partial cues, which serve as reminders. Recall is the active and unaided remembering of something from the past. Recognition refers to the ability to correctly identify previously encountered stimuli as familiar. Relearning may show evidence of the effects of memory; material that is familiar is often easier to learn a second time than it would be if it were unfamiliar.

The course of forgetting over time has been studied extensively by psychologists. Most often a rapid forgetting occurs at first, followed by a decreasing rate of loss. Improvement in the amount of material retained, however, can be achieved by practicing active recall during learning, by periodic reviews of the material, and by overlearning the material beyond the point of bare mastery. A mechanical technique devised to improve memory is mnemonics, involving the use of associations and various devices to remember particular facts. Four traditional explanations of forgetting have been provided. **One** is that memory traces fade naturally over time as a result of organic processes occurring in the nervous system, although little evidence for this notion exists. **A second** is that memories become systematically distorted or modified over time. **A third** is that new learning often interferes with or replaces old learning, a phenomenon known as retroactive inhibition. **Finally, some forgetting may be motivated by the needs and wishes of the individual, as in repression.**

Little is known about the physiology of memory storage in the brain. Some researchers suggest that memories are stored at specific sites, and others that memories involve widespread brain regions working together; both processes may in fact be involved. Theorists also propose that different storage mechanisms exist for short-term and long-term memories, and that if memories are not transferred from the former to the latter they will be lost. Animal studies indicate that structures in the brain's limbic system have different memory functions. For example, one circuit through the hippocampus and thalamus may be involved in spatial memories, whereas another, through the amygdala and thalamus, may be involved in emotional memories. Research also suggests that "skill" memories are stored differently from intellectual memories.

In general, memories are less clear and detailed than perceptions, but occasionally a remembered image is complete in every detail. This phenomenon, known as eidetic imagery, is usually found in children, who sometimes project the image so completely that they can spell out an entire page of writing in an unfamiliar language that they have seen for a short time.

Amnesia is perhaps the ultimate loss or impairment of memory. It may be caused by organic disorders, such as brain injury or cerebral arteriosclerosis, or by functional nervous disorders, such as hysteria. Amnesia may be total, with complete loss of recall; or partial, occurring only immediately before or after a traumatic event; or systematic, relating to a particular type or group of experiences. Amnesia is a symptom rather than a disease, and treatment attempts to determine and remove the basic cause.

The Brain Needs Six Hours ...

How long does it take for the brain to integrate and actually learn a new skill after practicing that new skill?

Brain researchers now believe the answer is six hours. After a person is shown, taught or practices a new skill, such as riding a bike or learning to cross-country ski, it takes about six hours for the brain to make a permanent record of that new skill. If the brain is interrupted by something else between the six hours of learning and integrating, the entire lesson may be lost, and the subject will have to start all over again.

The study was done at Johns Hopkins University. Scientists there said that time is a critical element in the process of learning. These researchers have concluded that it is not good enough to simply practice something, you must also allow a certain amount of time — about six hours — in which you do not move onto another equally complicated task.

All this was determined with the help of a device that measures blood flow in the brain, called a positron emission tomography machine, or PET for short. People were placed in the PET and then taught to manipulate an object on a computer screen by using motorized robot arm. The test required unusually precise and rapid hand movements that could be learned only through practice. The device indicated to researchers that new memories take five to six hours to move from temporary storage sites in the front of the brain to permanent storage sites located in the back of the brain.

But during that five or six hour time, the brain's memory system is vulnerable to easy erasure. If a second task of equal importance is taken up within before the brain has time to convert short term memory into long term memory, what is stored in the short term area of the brain will be dissolved in favor of the new. Scientists call this the "window of vulnerability."

For example, if a person spends an hour learning a tricky piano piece, and then immediately turns to a second difficult piece, they may undo all the hard work of learning the first! Therefore, it would be far better for the piano student to work hard on getting the first piece down, and then relax or engage in activities that do not require new learning skills for the next five or six hours.

Scientists called this information "a new and important clue about the relationship between motor-skill learning and neural activity."

Still, scientists admit that much more needs to be learned about how this all actually works. In other words, the 6-hour rule may not be an absolute that encompasses all learning skills all the time. In some instances, for example, the brain may use different parts of itself to learn one skill over another kind of skill. So a person may be able to learn swimming skills in one hour, and computer skills the next hour without one cancelling the other out. Swimming is a physical skill and learning computers involves memory and cognitive abilities, and are not closely related in terms of how the brain relates to each kind of activity.

During the PET examination stage of this research, the images obtained showed that blood flow was most active in the prefrontal cerebral cortex of the brain. After the learning session, the test subjects were allowed to do unrelated routine things for five to six hours and then were retested.

When operating the robot arm on the retest portion of the experiment, the blood flow was most active in the posterior parital and cerebella areas. Such a shift is necessary, scientists speculate, to protect the memory from being pushed aside by other input into the mind.

It is this very brain activity that allows a person to never forget a specific activity, such as riding a bike, or swimming.

Other subjects in this testing procedure were trained in a new motor task immediately after learning a new skill. Later, those subjects were tested on how much of the first lesson they could remember, only to discover that they had lost much of the original skill they had learned.

Scientists said this is strong evidence that teaching one task and immediately following it with a second task will erase the first, wasting a lot of time and effort.

The implications of this study are important and far reaching, if they turn out to be true. For example, are we planning lessons correctly in our school — that is, in such a way that allows the brains of students to properly absorb what they are being taught? Should students be allowed to study calculus one hour, and music the next. One class could be wiping out the other!

Having this kind of information about the learning process of the brain may revolutionize the way courses are laid out in school curriculums all over the world. And for those of you who are not in school, but who still enjoy learning new things, this information may be a powerful new tool for helping you learn new things more efficiently and with less frustration.

More Memory Muscle Builders

Memory is such an integral part of all aspects of thinking that boosting it alone will go a long way toward improving your overall ability to think clearly and be mentally alert. Perhaps nothing is associated with aging more than a failing memory. Fortunately, improving your memory is something that is easily done, and it doesn't take a doctor or thousands of dollars in high tech medical techniques to accomplish.

We are going to give your four fantastic ways to turn a weak and failing memory into an iron trap that never lets go of a single fact once it enters your brain for permanent storage.

Method 1: Mnemonic Tools and Acronyms

You all have undoubtedly used this technique at least once or twice some time during your life. This involves creating a word or sentence with each letter of that word or sentence standing for something you want to remember. For example, when you were in grammar school, you may have used A Rat In The House Might Eat The Ice Cream as a handy way to remember how to spell "arithmetic."

Sounds a bit trite and simple, but this technique is what helps thousands of doctors survive the rigors of medical school, where memorizing large volumes of complex materials is a must. For example, just one disease may have more than 100 possible medications which can be used for treatment.

Have you ever wondered why doctors rarely have to pick up a reference book to look up the name of a specific drug before they write your a prescription? It's because medical school requires they memorize hundreds, if not thousands, of drug names and what they should be used for. Doctors do that by word associations and acronyms to make the task possible.

If this technique works for everyone from school children to doctors, it certainly can work for you. Whether you want to memorize your shopping list, or remember all the names of your grandchildren, making up some kind of acronym to help you get the job done is an excellent idea.

Memory Method 2: Rhyming

In the ancient days before the invention of pen and paper to write things down, people had to rely much more heavily on their memories to retain large bodies of knowledge they needed to know. One of the primary ways they did it successfully was through use of rhymes.

Everyone knows the little trick for remembering how many days are in each of the 12 months: "Thirty days hath September, April, June and November, all the rest have 31 except February ..." Such an easy-to-remember rhyme makes the task a snap. You can apply this technique to just about anything you need to remember on a daily basis.

"I'll get ill if I don't take my pills."
"The day of the tenth is the day to pay my rent."
"My grandchild's name is Brent, and he was heaven sent."

Make a game out of it. Write down the things that are most vital for you to remember, such as when to take medication, when important bills are due, when your favorite TV show is on, and see if you can make up a cute little rhyme for each situation. You will not believe how easy this is, and how it turns your "ordinary" memory into a super-powered never-forgetting memory bank.

Memory Method 3: Visual Association

Some stage performers are really able to WOW their audiences by remembering extremely long lists of seemingly unrelated word items. They will ask audience members to create a random list of words: "chair, sky, zebra, tin can, book ..." and so on. They then repeat the list back, sometimes dozens of words long, purely from memory.

How do they do it? The trick is to make a visual association with each word, and link that visual image with each additional word. The more outrageous the visual image created, the better this technique works.

For example, in the the list given above, the person should form some kind of bizarre mental picture of a chair. Rather than just picturing an ordinary chair, the person should imagine something dramatic, such as a sizzling electric chair executing a prisoner, or the golden throne of God himself — they key it to form an extremely powerful image that is almost impossible to forget. Often, including painful or stressful or violent images is the best way to make a solid unforgettable image. A man frying in an electric chair may be horrible, but it is also hard to forget. Then go on to the next word, in this case sky. Picture the guy in the electric chair exploding and being sent into the wide blue sky above, and picture the electric chair turning into a kind of sky-writing airplane where it spells the word "sky" in puffy white smoke across a backdrop of perfect blue sky. Now you have two outrageous images which are linked together, and are almost impossible to forget!

Continue to create images — linked images — for each word in the list, and you will be able to perform seemingly fantastic feats of memory and recall that will absolutely amaze your friends.

This technique gets easier and more powerful the more you practice it and use it. In fact, some people get addicted to this form of memory building, simply because it is so fun and pleasurable!

Some scientists even speculate that the brain so much enjoys being worked and exercised in this way that it releases pleasure inducing hormones called endorphins into the blood stream. These endorphins create feeling of pleasure and satisfaction in people, even mild euphoria. Can doing something as simple as practicing mental exercises produce feelings of bliss and well-being? Apparently so!

Memory Method 4: Location Association

This is another memory tool which has been used for centuries by human beings as a way to remember large bodies of information without the use of lists or other mental crutches.

This method involves envisioning a place you know extremely well, such as your house with all it bedrooms and other rooms. Or it may be your neighborhood with all its streets or buildings.

What you do then is mentally "place" each item in a list of items you want to remember in each room or spot in the familiar landscape of your mind. For example, if you want to remember your grocery list, place a head of lettuce in the middle of the floor of your living room, a bottle of ketchup in the first bedroom, a pound of hamburger in the bathroom, a bag of noodles on the toilet seat, and so on.

The remembering process simply has you walking though your mental image and picking up each item as you move along. Once again, making each mental image as outrageous as possible will make this technique even more effective. For example, don't just place a head of lettuce in the middle of your living room carpet, place a head of lettuce the size of a baby elephant smack in the middle of your living room! It's hard to forget an image like that!!!

The most important element of all four of the methods above is using association. Memory is actually the process of recalling items we want to remember with a specific cue.

Once again, the more you practice these techniques, the better you get at them — and the brain responds by becoming stronger.

In fact, scientists have now proven that engaging in such mental exercises as we described above actually has the physical effects of building thicker and more numerous neuron branches within the brain. Just as muscles get thicker and stronger through lifting weights or some other form of exercise, running your brain through its paces will make it physically more massive, strong and thick with powerful neurons capable of a lot of mental heavy lifting.

Many people find using the above four methods cumbersome or difficult at first, but we can't emphasize enough the fact that improvement will come very quickly if you stick with it. Don't give up! Practice this method for just 15 to 20 minutes per day and you'll soon develop a super-powered memory that will be the envy of everyone you know.

A man or a woman with a powerful memory is a man or woman who has taken years off of his or her age. There is nothing like a sharp mind to give the appearance and the reality of youth.

Memory is not the only mental function which can be exercised to improve the overall health and ability of the brain. Another important factor in the thinking process is called cognition by psychologists and those who study the human brain.

Cognition is the act or process of knowing. Cognition includes attention, perception, memory, reasoning, judgment, imagining, thinking, and speech. Attempts to explain the way in which cognition works are as old as philosophy itself; the term, in fact, comes from the writings of Plato and Aristotle. With the advent of psychology as a discipline separate from philosophy, cognition has been investigated from several viewpoints.

An entire field of cognitive psychology has arisen since the 1950s. It studies cognition mainly from the standpoint of information handling. Parallels are stressed between the functions of the human brain and the computer concepts such as the coding, storing, retrieving, and buffering of information. The actual physiology of cognition is of little interest to cognitive psychologists, but their theoretical models of cognition have deepened understanding of memory, psycholinguistics, and the development of intelligence.

Social psychologists since the mid-1960s have written extensively on the topic of cognitive consistency — that is, the tendency of a person's beliefs and actions to be logically consistent with one another. When cognitive dissonance, or the lack of such consistency, arises, the person unconsciously seeks to restore consistency by changing his or her behavior, beliefs, or perceptions. The manner in which a particular individual classifies cognitions in order to impose order has been termed cognitive style.

Closely linked to cognition is intelligence itself. Intelligence is defined as the capacity to learn or to understand. It is generally synonymous with intellect but is usually differentiated from intellect in practice to emphasize ability or efficiency in dealing with concrete situations and in profiting intellectually from sensory experience. In psychology, intelligence is somewhat more narrowly defined as the capacity to acquire knowledge or understanding and to use it in novel situations. Under experimental conditions, the success of a subject in adjusting his or her behavior to the total situation or in meeting the challenge of the specific situation may be studied and, to some extent, measured in quantitative terms.

Psychologists believe that the capacities measured in testing or laboratory situations are also significant in everyday life, in which individuals analyze or apprehend new sensory and mental data so as to direct their actions toward desired goals. Psychologists still differ, however, as to a precise definition of the comprehensiveness and functions of intelligence; one school of thought considers it as a sum of specific abilities best displayed in specific situations.

In the formulation of intelligence tests, most psychologists tend to adopt an eclectic concept, according to which intelligence is treated as a general ability operating as a common factor in a wide variety of special aptitudes. It is observed and measured by techniques focused upon these aptitudes singly or in combination.

Improving Intelligence and Cognition

How do you improve intelligence and cognition? By using your brain to perform tasks which require intelligence and cognition! Just as memory grows stronger with more use of tasks that require memory, performing tasks which require critical thinking, cognition, intelligence, deductive thinking, use of strategy, problem solving and the rest will improve the functioning of the brain.

We have already mentioned that playing chess is an excellent way to improve overall memory cognition and intelligence. That because chess requires so much of the brain if it is going to be done well.

If you are a senior citizen, there are few better things you can do for your brain than to get together for a daily or twice a week chess match. This is the equivalent of going for a daily jog. Just as the jog whips your body into shape, a chess match will sprucc up the ability of your brain to work better in all aspects of life.

It doesn't have to be chess, as long as you pick an activity you both enjoy, and which requires heavy use of your mental faculties. Some examples are: working crossword puzzles, solving "brain twister" problems as presented in some books and magazines, or pursuing some other kind of intellectually oriented hobby or task that makes your life more rich and interesting.

If you read books, don't choose pulpy, trashy books, such as formulaic romance novels — read books that truly challenge your mind. Read books that have difficult concepts to understand, or topics that really make you grapple with what is being presented. Not every book you read has to make you sweat mental bullets. You may simply choose to include one difficult book for every five books of easy reading.

Just the act of reading itself, even if it is an easy book to read, is far better than spending hours a day engaging in activities that do not require much input from your own mind.

Without a doubt, the biggest and most damaging, brain rotting activity is watching television. Perhaps more than anything else, it is television which is destroying the brains of millions of our senior citizens today. The problem with television is that it does it all for you. You don't need to use your mind to form images when you can just passively stare at the TV screen which will spoon-feed images into your mind. You don't have to solve problems as you watch TV because the TV characters are engaged in solving the problems for you as a way to entertain you.

Television also destroys both memory and attention span. It does so by moving quickly from one image to the next, and doing so every few seconds. Television does not require you to focus on any one image or thought for more than 20 or 30 seconds at a time. Television producers long ago learned that the best TV shows are those that do not require a great deal of attention to enjoy. They know that a lot of people watch TV while doing other things, such as cleaning house, while talking to other people, or while there are a lot of other distractions around. Thus, the most successful TV shows are those with the most simple and thin plots, shows which require only a minimum of mental exertion by the viewer.

That may be a fine way for the mind to relax once and a while. But the problem is that most people watch several hours of television each and every day. Senior citizens are especially susceptible to being sucked in by the easy lure of television, especially if they are otherwise disabled and unable to go for walks or do other nonsitting activities they once used to enjoy.

The television, like a street corner drug pusher attracts unsuspecting victims with an almost impossible to resist array of mental candy — lights! camera! action! sound! sex! thrills! spills! adventure! comedy! laughs! — and all the rest.

Indeed, television acts very much like a drug to the mind. It makes people feel good, it puts them in a true altered state of consciousness, it is extremely addicting and it leads people away from other more productive and constructive activities of life.

In one interesting experiment, research psychologists got a group of parents to voluntarily take away television from their children, and then recorded the reaction of the group of children. As expected, the children displayed most of the same symptoms that alcoholics or drugs addicts experience when they are forced to withdraw from their booze or pills. The children became cranky and depressed. They started acting out, displaying anti-social, sometimes even violent behavior. They found themselves thinking about and craving their lost television, and fantasizing about ways to get it back.

Interestingly, after enough time passed without television, many of the children were able to kick their TV habit, and were amazed that they ever once spent so much time on something "so stupid and wasteful."

After just a week or two without television, most of the children began to show improvement in mood, were less hyperactive, calmer, and generally more interested and involved in "real life" activities. Once free from the drug of television, they realized how much time they had been wasting, and how much more vibrant life could be when they used their own minds to entertain themselves, rather than having a mindless television do it for them.

The point of all this is — to maintain a healthy and youthful brain well into the twilight years of our lives it is imperative that you keep your mind as active as possible with tasks that challenge the brain, and avoid those things which make things too easy on the brain — most dangerous of which is television.

Other Brain Killers

Maintaining a healthy mind also means avoiding those common substances which most medical researchers agree are harmful to the brain.

Perhaps the No. 1 brain killer in the world is alcohol. Alcohol is truly a "dumb drug." First of all, scientists have long suspected that alcohol actually kills brain cells, and otherwise causes the brain to deteriorate rapidly with age. Most of this belief is based on studies of the brains of life-time heavy drinkers, who almost always have less brain mass than people who have not drank heavily throughout their lives. Also, a disease known as organic brain syndrome, which is basically a drastic shrinking or deterioration of the brain, has long been suspected to be alcohol related.

Some researchers go as far as to say that every drink of alcohol kills several hundred thousand brain cells. Such a theory has never been proven, but there is no doubt that alcohol, at least in some complex way, contributes to the deterioration of the brain. In short, frequent drinking of alcohol is simply not compatible with a healthy, youthful mind well into the senior years.

Another certain brain killer is tobacco, and most specifically, cigarettes. Why are cigarettes so hard on the brain? Over time, cigarettes contribute heavily to the hardening of the arteries, including the arteries of the brain. In fact, smoking cigarettes contributes heavily to brain killing strokes, and not just major strokes, but most likely dozens of little minor strokes that may occur unnoticed — except for the fact that, little by little, they make the brain less efficient and confused.

Smoking cigarettes also restricts the flow of blood to the brain, depriving it of much needed oxygen. A brain deprived of oxygen is a brain that is unable to think at peak levels. A brain deprived of oxygen is also laid open to the ongoing damage of free radicals, which can break down the cells of the brains just as efficiently as they break down any other kind of cell in the human body.

Another possible source of danger to a healthy mind are artificial sweeteners, such as cyclamates, saccharin and aspartame, better known as Nutra Sweet. There is some scientific evidence to support the contention that NutraSweet can contribute to short-term memory loss, and possible long-term memory loss. Artificial sweeteners have also been linked to an increased number of
brain tumors among the general population. Thus, you may want to avoid soft drinks and other sweet foods that are made that way by aspartame or saccharin.

By the way, many medical researchers say it is a good idea to avoid all soft drinks because they come in aluminum cans. As we mentioned earlier, aluminum has been identified as a possible substance which causes damage to the brain.

In fact, the most dreaded form of senile dementia, Alzheimer's Disease, has been closely linked to increased amounts of aluminum in the human brain.

Learning and Genetics

A new study of Swedish twins who are 80 years of age or older shows that individual differences in how they acquire and process knowledge (cognition) relies as much on genetic inheritance patterns as on environmental factors.

The study is the first to look at the genetic influence (heritability) on many different aspects of cognition in older people, and confirms patterns that have emerged from similar studies in younger and middle-aged people. Because cognitive function plays a crucial role in determining the quality of life for older people, understanding how cognition develops as people age could lead to beneficial interventions that might slow or reverse cognitive decline.

A wide range of environmental variables such as geography, education, socioeconomic status, nutritional habits, occupation, disease and stress exposure might be expected to have substantial influences on cognition. Over the course of a lifetime, twins exposed to differing environments might be expected to display wide variances in cognition. Yet given the cumulative impact of a lifetime of environmental disparities, this study shows that the effects of environment on cognition are barely equal to the effects that genetic heritability has on cognition.

The research is unique in that it looks, in people age 80 and older, at general (intellectual ability) and specific (spatial, verbal, and memory) cognition, and examines in detail each of the 3 separate areas of specific cognition. Previous twin studies have shown that general cognitive abilities are among the most heritable behavior traits, with heritable influence increasing from 20 percent at infancy to 60 percent in adulthood. This finding contradicts the commonly held assumption that environmental influence increases throughout the life span with a corresponding decrease in genetic influence. The present study shows that the relative contributions of genetics and environment — about half and half — extends into very advanced age.

Investigators in this study were able to utilize the Swedish Twin Registry, which has tracked 96 percent of all twins in Sweden. The study utilized 240 sets of these twins born before the start of World War I. They were an average age of 83 years old. To assess cognitive abilities, twins were tested by licensed nurses using tests for verbal meaning, figure logic, block design, and picture memory. Analysis of combined scores of cognitive ability showed that heritability accounted for 55 percent of the individual differences in ability, a result similar to that seen in people who are middle-aged. The heritable impact on specific cognitive abilities, something little studied previously, was somewhat less than 50 percent but still highly significant.

For both general and specific cognitive abilities, identical twins, as would be expected, showed much stronger similarities than did fraternal twins. Additionally, living together or sharing the same environment in later life did not account for any significant similarity or dissimilarity of environmental impact on cognition.

It is now becoming possible to identify specific genes which may be responsible for some of the differences in cognitive abilities, researchers say. For example, certain forms of the ApoE gene have been associated with cognitive decline in older people, particularly in those with Alzheimer's disease.

Other researchers suggest the next step to better understanding genetic influences on cognition in older people is to conduct additional long-term studies on twins as well as studies using siblings and population-based samples. Discovering how we learn in old age could lead to a better understanding of how people can remain active and involved in society up to the very end of their lives.

Psychoactive Drugs

A discussion of a healthy, youthful brain could not be complete without a discussion of a powerful class of drugs called psychoactive drugs and their effect on the brain.

Psychoactive drugs are chemical substances that alter mood, behavior, perception, or mental functioning. Throughout history, many cultures have found ways to alter consciousness through the ingestion of substances. In current professional practice, psychoactive substances known as psychotropic drugs have been developed to treat patients with severe mental illness.

Psychoactive substances exert their effects by modifying biochemical or physiological processes in the brain. The message system of nerve cells, or neurons, relies on both electrical and chemical transmission. Neurons rarely touch each other; the microscopic gap between one neuron and the next, called the synapse, is bridged by chemicals called neuroregulators, or neurotransmitters. Psychoactive drugs act by altering neurotransmitter function. The drugs can be divided into six major pharmacological classes based on their desired behavioral or psychological effect: alcohol, sedative-hypnotics, narcotic analgesics, stimulant-euphoriants, hallucinogens, and psychotropic agents.

Alcohol has always been the most widely used psychoactive substance. In most countries it is the only psychoactive drug legally available without prescription. Pleasant relaxation is commonly the desired effect, but intoxication impairs judgment and motor performance. When used chronically, alcohol can be toxic to liver and brain cells and can be physiologically addicting, producing dangerous withdrawal syndromes.

Sedative-hypnotics, such as the barbiturates and diazepam (widely known under the brand name Valium), include brain depressants, which are used medically to help people sleep (sleeping pills), and antianxiety agents, which are used to calm people without inducing sleep. Sedative-hypnotics are used illegally to produce relaxation, tranquillity, and euphoria. Overdoses of sedative-hypnotics can be fatal; all can be physiologically addicting, and some can cause a life-threatening withdrawal syndrome.

Narcotic analgesic opiates such as morphine and heroin are prescribed to produce analgesia. Because the relief of pain is one of the primary tasks of medical treatment, opiates have been among the most important and valuable drugs in medicine. Illegal use of narcotic analgesics involves injecting these substances, particularly heroin, into the veins to produce euphoria. Opiates are physiologically addicting and can produce a quite unpleasant withdrawal syndrome.

Stimulant-euphoriants, such as amphetamines, are prescribed by physicians to suppress the appetite and to treat children often diagnosed as hyperactive. Although amphetamines stimulate adults, they have a paradoxically calming effect on certain children who have short attention spans and are hyperactive. Cocaine is used medically as a local anesthetic. Amphetamines and cocaine are used illegally to produce alertness and euphoria, to prevent drowsiness, and to improve performance in physical and mental tasks such as athletic events and college examinations.

Hallucinogens or psychedelic drugs such as LSD, mescaline, and PCP thus far have little medical use. They are taken illegally to alter perception and thinking patterns. Marijuana is a weak hallucinogen that may be medically useful in suppressing the nausea caused by cancer treatments and possibly in reducing eye pressure in certain severe glaucomas.

Psychotropic drugs have been in use since the early 1950s. Antipsychotic drugs decrease the symptoms of schizophrenia, allowing many schizophrenic patients to leave the hospital and rejoin community life. Antidepressant drugs help the majority of patients with severe depression recover from their disorder. Lithium salts eliminate or diminish the episodes of mania and depression experienced by manic-depressive patients.

NOTES

_____

_____

_____

_____

_____

_____

_____

_____

_____

Chapter 11

Special Report:
Smart Drugs and the
Chemistry of Mental Youth

Tomorrow is an extremely important day for you. You are going to that big job interview, and you are trying to land the high-paying "dream job" you have worked for years to achieve. Sure, you're what most people would call a senior citizen. Yes, this new job represents a second career for you. But so what? You want this job as bad as any up-and-coming 28 year old. If you can do the job as well or better than any other candidate, age should be a none factor.

Right now, you are concentrating on being in tip-top mental form for your interview. You want to be as sharp as a newly minted razor blade. You can't let anything get you down — your age, your energy level, a flagging memory, an inability to think on your feet and be alert.

Even though you are already in superb shape — you have replenished the hormones in your body back to their youthful levels, you have brought your body back into peak fitness with regular, rigorous exercise, you have kept your mind active and applied after your first "retirement" — is there anything more you can do?

Yes! You can take a trip to the drug store!

What you want to do is "fine-tune" the biochemistry of your brain. You want to create the optimal neurochemical conditions for creativity, cognition and peak mental performance.

So you ask the pharmacist for some pointers. He then guides you to the shelf of the latest mind enhancement supplements. You fill up your basket with bottles of such compounds as piracetam, vasopressin, hydergine, choline, DMAE, and maybe a little centrophenoxine.

At home you take the directed doses of each. Then you retire to your study where you slip on your cranial electric simulator along with your light and sound device — your very own portable mind tune-up machine.

The combination of the supplements and your mind machine balance your brain in a way that puts you into peak mental and psychological shape, meaning you can be at your very best exactly when you need to be.

After an hour with your mind machine, and after your brain supplements have had a time to work their way into your blood stream you feel extremely relaxed, yet creative, mentally sharp — ready for anything. **Your brainwave activity has changed.** An electronic measurement of your brainwave patterns would reveal a more regular pattern. Your test would show an increase in amplitude in certain frequencies, causing you to feel simultaneously profoundly relaxed yet in a state of intense concentration, loose and creative as well as mentally quick and alert.

Furthermore, a brain-mapping device would show that the two hemispheres of your brain were in a state of "super connection," with an enormous increase in the amount of information flowing between the hemispheres. At the same time, the rate of metabolism and the energy level of your brain cells have sharply increased. You are now in the optimal state to imprint new memories, to plan new and more creative strategies, to visually rehearse every detail of your upcoming interview.

Do you think all this sounds like some far-off scenario of some science fiction movie?

Well, the truth of the matter is that both the brain machines and the cognitive enhancement compounds are already available to anyone in the market.

In just the past few years, a whole family of mind-magnifying drugs have emerged on the market, as well as droves of solid evidence of their ability to amplify learning, memory and thinking. What we don't know is how to best use them together, or even whether they should be used together. That's what we want to find out. The problem, as many of you are aware, is that it is extremely difficult for those interested in performing research into the effects of brain machines to obtain the necessary funding and support.

Mainstream science, particularly those elements in control of doling out grants and funds to support research, and many of the universities and institutions engaged in research, seem to have little interest in investigating mind machines, used in combination with brain enhancing supplements.

That research which is performed usually involves the therapeutic applications of the devices rather that the induction of peak performance brain states. On the other hand, huge amounts of money are being spent for research into cognition enhancing drugs. But much of the research is being done by the big pharmaceutical companies, who are racing with each other to develop patentable memory enhancement drugs and to obtain FDA approval for these compounds.

Because the FDA is focused on treating diseases in a medical context and has not shown much interest in giving its approval to drugs that simply improve people's memories or boost intelligence, the pharmaceutical companies are directing their efforts toward gaining approval for their cognition-enhancement drugs as treatments for medical problems such as Alzheimer's disease, multiple-infarct dementia and senility.

Because financial analysts estimate that such cognitive drugs could quickly produce sales of well over a billion dollars a year in the U.S. alone, and ultimately outsell antibiotics and tranquilizers, the competition is fierce, and these companies are in no mood to investigate ways their substances might work in cooperation with other substances or other mechanisms such as mind machines.

Also, since their efforts are directed toward drugs that are patentable, these companies have little interest in exploring the cognition enhancement properties of substances that cannot be patented. Vitamin C is a good example: In a controlled study in which healthy individuals were tested both for levels of vitamin C and IQ, those with higher levels of the vitamin averaged 5 points higher in IQ; when those with the lower levels of the vitamin were given vitamin C supplements, their IQ scores increased by more than 3.5 points.

In some way, vitamin C is a cognition-enhancing substance. But, of course no one can patent vitamin C, which is cheap and readily available. In another example, one widely available and unpatentable substance (DHEA) is rumored to have demonstrated in a recent study some success in, among other things, treating AIDS, as well as cognition enhancement; however, the drug company involved in the experiments is now apparently trying to conceal the discoveries about DHEA until it can develop some variant that is patentable, and has obtained a court order forbidding the scientist in charge of the study to even speak with anyone about the matter.

Still, at this point, it is probably too dangerous to go out and take large quantities of the substances we have already mentioned in this chapter. High level mental functioning can be exceedingly dangerous and have frightening and unpredictable side effects.

Nevertheless, it will be interesting here to outline what lies on the cutting edge of mind/brain enhancement, in terms of boosting the intelligence of the human mind, no matter how old or how young.

First let's describe a few of the most promising cognition enhancing substances.

Memory Enhancing Drugs

The drug, physostigmine, when administered to people by infusion in laboratory tests, aids and improves performance of everyday working memory. Working memory is the process which temporarily holds information such as a phone number until a person gets to a phone to dial the number.

In a new laboratory study, conducted at the National Institute on Aging (NIA), researchers used positron emission tomography (PET) to find and monitor the areas of the human brain that are activated during working memory, and to determine how activity in those regions is modified by a working memory enhancing drug.

Physostigmine is a short-acting drug that enhances levels of a substance (acetylcholine) between neurons in the brain. The drug improves efficiency and reduces the effort needed to perform working memory tasks while altering the activity of some of the brain regions activated by this memory task.

Scientists point out that during the brief period the investigators monitored brain activity, the volunteers' abilities to recognize faces they had just been shown were improved when given the test drug. Furey continues, "A better understanding of how working memory functions could give us valuable clues as to how our brains process and manipulate such information. It could also teach us about how drugs that alter some cognitive processes, such as working memory, influence the brain's response."

Tacrine, the first approved drug for treatment against Alzheimer's disease, acts on the acetylcholine system in a way similar to physostigmine. Dr. Furey believes that since physostigmine improved the brain's response to memory tasks (which are related to observed improvements in performance), similar drugs that enhance the cholinergic system might help relieve symptoms in Alzheimer's disease patients. For now, however, tacrine is a more practical drug to use clinically to relieve the symptoms of Alzheimer's disease since it is longer-acting than this form of physostigmine.

To conduct their study, Dr. Furey and colleagues recruited volunteers to NIA laboratories for a series of ten PET scans. The volunteers were separated into control and experimental groups which were matched by age, education, and gender. The ten PET scans allowed researchers to identify the areas of the brain where activity was taking place. The scans alternated between resting and memory task assignments. During the task scans for each trial, volunteers were shown a picture of a person's face, followed by a brief delay period during which subjects had to retain the information, followed by a test condition where subjects had to select from two faces, one of which they had seen earlier. The faces were then changed for each subsequent trial. The control volunteers received only saline during their brain scans whereas the experimental volunteers received physostigmine. Drug levels were checked after each scan by taking blood samples.

PET scan results were then evaluated to identify those areas of the brain that were active during working memory to determine how the two conditions differed, both with and without physostigmine.

The results of the trials showed that enhancing acetylcholine transmission with physostigmine resulted in improved working memory performance and altered neural activity in a cortical region known to be important to this memory task. Pietro Pietrini, M.D., NIA scientist and another author of the study, points out that the mechanisms by which physostigmine acts remain unclear.

The drug may enhance efficiency during the processing of information by focusing attention on the task at hand or it could help minimize the effects of distracting stimuli. Either way, a more efficient working memory could be a great advantage for Alzheimer's disease patients and other memory-impaired people. Pietrini points out that the NIA is currently involved in a more in-depth analysis of working memory using a different imaging technique (functional MRI) that he hopes will lead us to an even better understanding of this intriguing aspect of brain function.

Beyond Memory: Cognitive Enhancing, or Nootropic Drugs

PIRACETAM

This is a drug which has been the subject of intensive research for over 15 years and has not only proven to be a powerful intelligence booster and cerebral stimulant, but also, even in massive acute and chronic dosages, appears to be nontoxic and to produce no side effects (it's so nontoxic one FDA employee reportedly claimed that since huge doses produce no toxic effects, it can't possibly have any pharmacological effects and must be physiologically inert). It is so remarkable in its effects and safety that its discovery by UCB Laboratories in Belgium sent virtually every other major pharmaceutical company scrambling to develop its own cerebral stimulant. This "Smart pill race" has resulted in the creation of a new drug category called the nootropics, from the Greek words noos (mind) and tropein (turn), meaning "acting on the mind."

Some of nootropic drugs being tested now on humans include vinpocetine (being developed by Ayerst Laboratories), which researchers believe speeds up learning, improves memory and recall and seems to block the action of substances that disrupt memory; an iracetam, which appears to be about ten times more potent in improving and protecting memory than piracetam, pramiracetam, which seems to improve learning and memory by enhancing the firing of neurons in the hippocampus (a key to the formation of long-term memories), andoxiracetam, apparently two to three times as powerful as pirac-

etam (intriguingly, research shows that when oxirac-
etam is given to pregnant rats their off spring proved
more intelligent that control groups—similar findings have been reported for the offspring of pregnant
rats kept in "enriched environments.

All of these substances seem remarkably nontoxic
and free of side effects. As yet, there is no nootropic
drug that is approved by the FDA for sale in the US,
but, keenly aware of the multi-billion dollar potential
of nootropics, the drug companies are pouring big
bucks into research that will satisfy FDA requirements by proving how they work (still not well
understood), and by proving their effectiveness in
treating medical problems such as Alzheimer's
disease and senility.

Piracetam has been proven to boost learning and
memory in normal subjects as well as those who suffer cognitive deficits, and is also a cognitive
enhancer under conditions of hypoxia, or too little
oxygen, which would make it an excellent substance
to pack along on a hike into the mountains.

A variety of clinical studies with human subjects,
including studies of young healthy volunteers,
healthy middle-aged subjects with some memory
decline, elderly subjects, elderly subjects with senility, and alcoholics, have proven that piracetam
enhances cortical vigilance, improves integration of
information processing, improves attention span
and concentration, and can produce dramatic
improvements in both direct and delayed recall of
verbal learning.

It's effective in the treatment of dyslexia, stroke, alcoholism, vertigo, senile dementia, sickle-cell anemia, and many other conditions, enhances the brain's resistance to various injuries and boosts its ability to recover from injuries, protects the brain against chemicals such as barbiturates and cyanides, and is widely used throughout Europe and Latin America (where it is sold over the counter).

The subjective effect described by a lot of people is that it "wakes up your brain." In fact, it selectively stimulates the anterior or frontal part of the forebrain—that part of the brain that has evolved most recently, rapidly and remarkably in the course of our evolution from ape to human, and which is the seat of our "higher functions."

Piracetam works in a number of ways to increase energy within the brain. First, it steps up the production of adenosinetriphosphate (ATP), the energy storage and energy generating molecules within our cells. It also boosts cerebral metabolism by improving cerebral microcirculation (blood flow), increasing the brain's use of glucose, and increasing the brain's oxygen use.

It also seems to enhance protein syntheses in the brain (it's been proven that protein synthesis is an essential step in laying down long-term memories).

Superconnecting the Brain

Perhaps the most intriguing aspect of piracetam is that it has been proven to increase the flow of information between the right and left hemispheres of the brain. As a result of experiments with human subjects one researcher concluded that piracetam causes the hemispheres to become "superconnected."

Since there's increasing evidence that high level brain states—brilliance, insight, creativity, flow, peak performance, being "in the zone"—are a product of the integrated and synergistic functioning of both hemispheres simultaneously, we might suspect that piracetam enhances not only simple learning and memory but creative or syntheses thinking.

Piracetam's capacity to superconnect the hemispheres becomes even more intriguing in light of the evidence indicating that many of the most widely used mind machines and techniques for brain enhancement function in part by facilitating integrated hemispheric functioning.

This raises the possibility that since both the machines and piracetam seem to facilitate interhemispheric communication, there might be a potentiating or synergistic effect when such mind machines are used in combination with piracetam, resulting in a quantum leap in brain-enhancement effects.

Precautions

Piracetam may increase the effects of certain drugs, such as amphetamines and psychotropics. Adverse effects are rare but include insomnia, psychomotor agitation, nausea, headaches and gastrointestinal distress.

Dosage

Piracetam is supplied in 400mg or 800mg tablets. The usual dose is 2400-4800 mg per day in three divided doses. Some literature recommends that for the first two days high "attack" doses should be taken. When some people first take piracetam they do not notice any effect until they take a high dose. Thereafter, they may notice that a lower dosage is sufficient. The drug takes effect in 30 to 60 minutes.

Sources

Piracetam is not sold in the US. It can be purchased over the counter in Mexico or by mail order from the address below.

Hydergine

A wealth of research going back over 20 years suggests that Hydergine may be what psychologist-pharmacist Ross Pelton calls "the ultimate smart pill." The substance, whose generic name is ergoloid mesylates, is made from a natural, organic source: the ergot fungus of rye plants (it was discovered at Sandoz laboratories by the visionary chemist Dr. Albert Hofmann.)

It increases mental abilities, prevents damage to brain cells, and may even be able to reverse existing damage to brain cells. Hydergine acts in several ways to enhance mental capabilities and to slow down or reverse the aging processes in the brain.

A few of the huge number of beneficial effects scientists have attributed to Hydergine include:

increased protein syntheses in the brain; reduced accumulation of lipofuscin in the brain; increased quantities of blood and oxygen delivered to the brain; improvement of memory, learning and intelligence; beneficial improvements in brainwave activity; increased metabolism in brain cells; normalization of blood pressure; and increased production of such neurotransmitters as dopamine and norepinephrine (neurochemical messengers essential to the formation of memory and also associated with arousal, alertness, elation and pleasure).

Hydergine also functions as a powerful antioxidant and thus protects the brain against the damage caused by those infamous rascally free radicals (unstable and extremely reactive molecules produced by normal metabolism, which cause damage associated with aging, cancer and cardiovascular disease).

One way that Hydergine may enhance brain functioning is by mimicking the effect of a substance called nerve growth factor (NGF). NGF promotes the growth of dendrites—the long branching fibers by which neurons receive information from other neurons. Scientists studying the effects of learning on the brain have found it is directly related to dendritic growth. Hydergine seems to work by the same neurochemical pathway as NGF to produce neural growth.

While Hydergine is widely used for the treatment of senility, scientists have also studied its effects, both short term and long term, in normal healthy humans; these studies noted significant improvements in a variety of cognitive function, including alertness, memory, reaction time, abstract reasoning and cognitive processing ability.

Precautions

If too large a dose is used when first taking Hydergine, it may cause slight nausea, gastric disturbance, or headache. Overall, Hydergine does not produce serious side effects, it is non-toxic even at very large doses, and it is contraindicated only for individuals who have chronic or acute psychosis.

Dosage

The U.S. recommended dosage is 3mg per day, however, the European recommended dosage is 9 mg per day taken in three divided doses. Most of the research has been done at levels of 9 to 12 mg per day or higher, and there is some evidence that 3 mg per day is simply insufficient for significant cognition-enhancement effects. It may take several weeks or even months before Hydergine produces noticeable effects. Hydergine (though not its generic counterpart) is available in a sublingual form, and there is evidence that sublingual doses reach the brain in greater quantity.

Sources

Hydergine is available in the U.S.A. with a doctor's prescription and approved by the FDA for the treatment of senile dementia and insufficient blood circulation to the brain. Your doctor may not be familiar with the uses discussed. It can also be purchased over the counter in Mexico or by mail order from overseas. In many cases these mail order companies sell the generic form, Ergoloid Mesylates. The FDA has rated the generic as biologically equivalent to the Sandoz product. More testing needs to be done on the question.

Vasopressin

Vasopressin, called "the memory hormone," is a natural brain peptide, stimulated by acetylcholine and released in the pituitary. It actually helps create, imprint, and store memories and is essential to remembering.

Apparently vasopressin is involved in picking out and chunking together related bits of information from the stream of consciousness, integrating these chunks into coherent structures, and then "imprinting" these images or concepts into long-term memory by transforming electrical impulses into complex proteins that contain memories and are stored away in the brain. The act of remembering the stored information is also mediated by vasopressin.

More than 20 years ago scientists discovered that vasopressin had extraordinary effects on the memory of laboratory animals—preventing chemically and electrically induced amnesia, actually reversing amnesia, and dramatically boosting the memory and intelligence of normal animals. These findings spurred much research into the cognition-enhancement effect of vasopressin on humans.

Among the key findings are that small doses of the hormone can have striking success in quickly reversing traumatic amnesia (amnesia caused by injuries such as car crashes), can reverse age-related memory loss and actually restore lost memories, and can produce sharp improvements in learning and memory using measures such as abstract and verbal memory, organizational capacities, recall, attention, concentration, focus, short-term memory, optical memory, and long-term memory.

It also boosts performance in such areas as reaction speed, visual discrimination, and coordination. Vasopressin pours out during moments of trauma or extreme arousal, which may explain why those times seem to be so deeply imprinted in our brains, and are remembered with such clarity. Vasopressin is also released by cocaine, LSD, amphetamines, Ritalin, and Pemoline (Cylert).

Those who make frequent use of these drugs deplete their brain's vasopressin supply. The result is depression and a decline in cognitive function. The frequent user's response to this depression is to take more of the drug, thus trying to wring more vasopressin out of their depleted brain: ultimately the well runs dry.

Vasopressin, however, is not a drug but the actual brain hormone that has been depleted, so it can produce dramatic and virtually instantaneous improvements in mood and mental functioning. Unlike stimulants, alcohol and marijuana do not deplete but actually suppress the release of vasopressin, which could account for the loss of memory many have noticed when drunk or stoned, or when trying to remember events that occurred while they were high.

Vasopressin can reduce the harmful effects of these drugs and enhance alertness, reaction speed and concentration. Anecdotal evidence suggests that vasopressin can produce a state of euphoria accompanied by self-confidence, energy, assertiveness, and a sensation of extreme mental clarity.

Many believe it is ideal for situations in which lots of new information needs to be processed and remembered—such as studying for an exam, learning a language, ploughing through difficult or complex works. Some use it for more mundane purposes, such as when they have to drive late at night and want to remain alert.

Precautions

Vasopressin can occasionally produce the following side effects; runny nose, nasal congestion, irritation of the nasal passages, headache, abdominal cramps, and increased bowel movements. Angina sufferers should not use vasopressin, since it can trigger angina pains. Vasopressin has not been proven to be safe for use during pregnancy.

Dosage

Vasopressin usually comes in a nasal spray bottle. Most studies showing memory improvement have been done with a dose of 12 to 16 USP per day, which is one whiff in each nostril three to four times per day. Vasopressin produces a noticeable effect within seconds.

Sources

Vasopressin (known as Diapid and produced by Sandoz) is available in the U.S.A. with a doctor's prescription, but keep in mind that your doctor may not be familiar with the uses we have discussed (it is approved by the FDA for treatment of diabetesinsipidus). It can also be purchased over the counter in Mexico or by mail order from overseas.

While some of the substances described above are not available in the U.S. or are available only by prescription, it is easy and quite legal to obtain these substances by mail order. One reason some of these substances are not available in the U.S. is that they have not yet gone through the extraordinarily expensive and lengthy process required to obtain FDA approval. This does not mean however that it is not quite legal to use these substances. And some of the substances have been approved by the FDA for limited medical application. This does not mean that it is not quite proper to use these substances for "unapproved" purposes.

In the April, 1982 issue of the FDA Drug Bulletin, the agency included a policy statement clarifying the question of "unapproved" uses for drugs, clearly stating that " 'unapproved' uses may be appropriate and rational in certain circumstances, and may, in fact, reflect approaches to drug therapy that have been extensively reported in medical literature. Valid new uses for drugs already on the market are often first discovered through serendipitous observations and therapeutic innovation."

In sum, the FDA clearly approves of the "unapproved" uses as an important means for innovation and discovery. Also, though it is not widely known, a July, 1989 FDA ruling now makes it quite legal to import effective drugs used elsewhere but not available in the U.S. The FDA now allows the importation and mail shipment of a three-month supply of drugs, for personal use, as long as they are regarded as safe in other countries.

The new ruling, FDA pilot guidelines chapter 971, was made as a result of heavy pressure from AIDS political action groups, which insisted AIDS sufferers were denied access to potentially life-saving substances that were widely used abroad but were still unapproved for use in the U.S. In Home Health Services, a mail order pharmacy in Switzerland, is one of a number of companies established in response to this new FDA ruling. In Home carries a wide variety of drugs for cognitive enhancement, life extension, and the treatment of AIDS which are not available in the US. All of the drugs discussed here can be purchased without a prescription.

Plant Products

They form the basis of most smart drinks, with or without amino acids. Many of these products are available in South Africa from health food shops.

- Guerana provides an energy boost similar to caffeine, but has a slower and more lasting effect.

- Kava-kava has a calming, relaxing effect.

- Ginseng is said to have "life-enhancing" qualities.

- Pausinystata is derived from the bark of a West African tree and is said to be used in two-week long sex ceremonies!

- Long-Sha is a Chinese herb traditionally used as a food supplement.

- Ma Huang, also Chinese, used as a brain stimulant.

AMINO ACIDS

Essential nutrients, used in many smart drinks.

- L-Phenylalanine releases noradrenaline, which improves one's mood.

- L-Pyroglutamic acid occurs naturally in brain fluids.

Other amino acids are protein components.

OTHER NUTRIENTS

Used in smart drinks, widely available from pharmacies and health shops.

- Antioxidants such as vitamins A, C and E protect brain cells from damage.

- B vitamins have positive effects on the nervous system.

- Choline and Lecithin are turned by your body into acetylcholine, which transmits neural impulses in the brain.

Chapter 12

Mind over Matter:
How to Think Yourself Young

This chapter will be different from all the rest in this book, but it may very well be the most important. That's because it will approach the subject of youth renewal from the perspective of mind, rather than biology.

For those of you whose immediate reaction is to flip ahead to the next chapter, we urge you to reconsider. For those of you who are more interested in pills, patches or powders that will take away all your ills and keep you young, you should be warned that all the newest miracle substances may have no effect on your physical body if your "mental body" has not been programmed to go along for the ride, so to speak.

Most advice in medical books and self-help books focus on biological and physiological factors that affect the human body, and tell about drugs, foods or techniques which can be used to achieve longer life.

Unfortunately, we as a society and as individuals too often try to adjust and manipulate the physical body as if it were a machine that could be made to run more efficiently if only the right ingredients can be found and added to it in the just the right amounts. Indeed, this may be the case, as we have seen in our thorough examination of superhormones and other substances which can balance the biochemistry of the body.

The fact that the mind — along with human emotions, beliefs and attitudes — has a direct connection and cannot be disputed. The following study is a significant reminder of that.

Scientists at the University of Goteborg in Sweden took a random sample of 50-year-old men and gave them each a physical examination and psychological evaluation. Seven years later, the researchers went back to find the men, and also looked up those who had died. What they found was that, of the men who had reported three or more recent upsetting events in their lives, 11 percent were dead. All of them identified themselves as lacking family or social support.

Of the men who had peaceful lives full of friends and family, just three percent had died.

The life events most strongly related to dying were having serious concerns about a family member, being forced to move, feelings of insecurity at work, serious financial trouble and being the target of legal action.

Swedish scientists think that stress may lower resistance to disease, and that lack of caring, loving people in your life provides less psychological "will" to fight off disease and to go forward with life.

Therefore, to significantly increase your chances of living longer, take a look at your own life. Do you have a family? a close friend, or friends? If you don't, perhaps now is the time to open yourself up to the possibility.

But the larger point is that, as the above story demonstrates, the aging of the body has a strong connection to the mind and the level of happiness or unhappiness of the individual. The Swedish study points to tantalizing clues which lead toward the conclusion that adjustments of the psychological aspect of life can an enormous effect on what happens to the physical body.

Another bit of scientific evidence also supports this claim, and we have already touched on this in the chapter on DHEA. We're talking about the study which showed that people who meditate can actually make their body produce larger amounts of DHEA in the bloodstream.

As reported in a recent issue of the "Journal of Behavioral Medicine," people who meditate on a regular basis have levels of age-related hormones that are comparable to those of meditators five to 10 years younger.

In the study, the level of DHEA of 423 meditators were compared to that of 1,252 healthy nonmeditators. The subjects were divided into groups according to their age, and meditators were compared to nonmeditators in the same age proximity.

Meditating females showed higher DHEA levels than nonmeditating women in every age group. Men under age 40 showed little variation, but after age 40, meditators began to show significantly higher levels of the youth hormone than nonmeditators.

So to be complete, one must consider that all the remedies and additives may be insignificant next to some important adjustments which people can make in their own mind.

Since we have already seen that scientific studies prove that meditation helps keep you young, the following is a meditation technique you can start practicing right away.

Meditating for Youth Renewal

There are perhaps as many ways to meditate as there are people who practice this mental and physical discipline, which bestows almost unlimited health benefits on those who use it regularly.

Since this is a book devoted to the topic of staying young, we'll look at some simple meditation techniques you can practice for just 5 to 10 minutes per day that will yield tremendous benefits to your mental and physical well-being, and which will slow the clock of time and its effects on your body.

First, a couple of facts about meditation that may make you feel more comfortable with it.

Meditation is not necessarily a religious exercise. It is not associated exclusively with eastern religions, such as Zen Buddhism, the Sufi sects of Islam, the Yogi masters of India, or others. Meditation is not something only people involved in cults or esoteric eastern religions do. There are many forms of Christian meditation, as well as meditation techniques that have nothing to do with religion what so ever.

Just because you decide to practice meditation does not mean you have to abandon your current religion, nor does it mean you are doing anything that is "weird" or somehow philosophically unwholesome.

Meditation is safe for anyone to practice. Meditation does not involve going into a trance, or putting yourself in a state of mind that will make you passive, or open to unwanted mental intrusions from negative sources. Meditation also does not involve sitting in an uncomfortable, contorted position on the floor, burning incense or chanting — unless you choose to do those things. **Simply put, meditation merely involves sitting quietly, clearing your mind of troubles and turmoil, and seeking a feeling of peace and being centered...**

How to meditate

So now that we have done away with some of the myths of meditation, let's try it out.

Meditation can be incredibly simple, yet deceptively difficult at times. The whole trick of meditation (if there is a trick at all) is to sit or lie down quietly and release everything from your mind, whether it be positive or negative thoughts.

Try this:

Find a chair in a quiet room where there are no other people, no television or radio playing and no other distractions.

Sit in your chair, but don't sit like you usually do. Sit closer to the edge of the chair. Put your feet flat on the floor, and keep your back straight. Put your hands palms down on your knees. You should be able to draw a straight line from the bottom of your spine, up through your back, neck and the back of your head — and the line would be perpendicular with the ceiling.

Don't try to be too stiff, as if a metal rod has been rammed down your spine. Just keep yourself generally straight, as if your were trying to practice good posture.

The next thing you want to do is take three slow, deep breaths. As you inhale imagine that you are drawing positive energy into your body, and as you exhale, imagine that all pain and negativity is rushing out of your body. Do it anyway you want. Some people like to imagine a stream of golden, positive energy entering their body as they inhale, and black or gray negative energy leaving their body as they exhale. But it's really up to you how you want to visualize this. It's usually best to invent your own way.

After doing three big breaths, you will probably notice that your mind is more quiet and more focused, that your heart rate is more steady, and you are feeling more calm.

The next thing you want to do is to simply see how long you can maintain this peaceful mental state, concentrating on your breathing, and keeping your mental activity to a minimum. The first day, try for 5 minutes and eventually work your way up to 10 minutes per session.

An important tip: Don't try too hard to keep your mind clear and calm. The harder you try, the more difficult you will find it to keep your mind empty.

You will find that all kinds of thoughts will persistently intrude on your attempt to remain calm and empty. It's incredibly difficult to let go of the million things we all have to think about each day — but that's the whole purpose of meditation — to give yourself a break from the daily chatter in your mind.

Don't worry, it's only for ten minutes. You can go back to whatever thoughts or worries you wish after your meditation session has been completed. But for just this ten minutes, once per day, commit yourself to a calm mind.

And at this point you might be thinking: How could anything so simple and uncomplicated really do me any good, especially for only 5 to 10 minutes per day?

But the facts are — and there is an enormous amount of medical data to back this up — that meditation can do everything from lower your blood pressure, to cure cancer, heal your heart, lower your cholesterol level, ease your addictions and much more.

Meditation is widely regarded by those inside and outside the medical community as one of the most powerful tools available for both preventative health care and for easing existing conditions.

Because most of our lives are so fast-paced and so filled with endless stress and activities, the precious ten minutes you give yourself once a day may be the very oasis of sanity that will allow your body to catch up and strengthen itself against the daily onslaught of the fast-paced American lifestyle, which most of us face everyday.

To sum up:

To meditate you need to remember only four basic things:

1) Find a quite, undisturbed place where you can be alone for 10 minutes without distractions.

2) Sit in a comfortable, upright posture, with back straight and face forward, hands on your knees. You may also lie flat on your back with hands at your sides or on your stomach.

3) Concentrate on your breathing while ignoring all your other thoughts. Note: It is extremely important that you don't try to "fight off" your thoughts. This will only make them louder and more persistent. Just let them run past you — let your mind flow like a stream, a stream which you pay little attention to.

4) Do it at least once a day, although a ten-minute session in the morning and an equal one at night will bring optimum results.

You've done it!

That's all there is to it! If you practice this simple meditation once or twice a day, you may start noticing results in your daily life and general level of health immediately. If you don't get immediate results, stick with it for two weeks. If by then you can still say meditation has done you no good, then you've wasted little time, and you'll know this stuff is not for you.

The Power of Visualization

Now we want to direct your attention to another powerful tool of the mind and its ability to wrestle away control of your physical body from Mother Nature, giving it back to you. **It's called visualization.** As its name suggests, visualization is the process of creating an image in your mind for the purposes of making that image a reality in your life.

What is Visualization?

Simply put, visualization involves putting the human body and mind into a deeply relaxed state and then forming a specific image in the mind in an extremely focused and detailed way.

The more a person practices this, the more control he or she develops over their own mind, and the object or thing being visualized. Visualizing a single object helps a person develop a certain one-pointedness of mind. This leads to a heightened state of alertness, clear thinking, and identification with the object being visualized.

Visualization does not have to involve focus on an object. One can also visualize a specific state of being or action that you would like to make a reality. For example, a person who is obese may want to visualize themselves as being skinny, or as being at some optimum weight level. A person who is poor and living on welfare can visualize a life of being wealthy and surrounded by all the good things in life. A person who is weak, frail and sickly, can visualize themselves as being in excellent robust health.

The point is to bring whatever it is that you visualize into your life, and bringing it from the point of being something in your mind to the point of having that thing exist in actual reality.

For the purposes of this book, we are interested in visualizing ourselves as young healthy people, no matter what our current age or our current state of health. Basically, we're talking about thinking ourselves young. If you are skeptical this can be done, and if you think visualization is all a lot of New Age nonsense, we think that you should reconsider.

A Brief History of Visualization

In just the past few decades, hundreds of doctors, scientists and ordinary individuals have been "discovering" the enormous power and potential of visualization, but the more proper term should be "rediscovering. That's because visualization is one of the most ancient practices known to civilized human beings.

If we go back to a time before humans were civilized, we can already see that ancient peoples were practicing visualization right from the beginning. Archeologists have discovered hundreds of cave paintings around the world which depict wild animals, along with depictions of human beings hunting those wild animals for food and to make items of clothing and weapons. Scientists believe these cave paintings were a form of visualization. By forming a strong image of what they wanted in their minds, and solidifying those images by actually putting them down on rock with paint and brush, the hunters were able to draw what they wanted to themselves in real life.

This is interesting because just about all of our modern day self-help gurus suggest setting goals by first thinking of what you want, and then writing it all down on paper as a way to solidify your goals and to make sure you achieve them. There is something about writing your goals down on paper that gives them a greater reality and solidity, making it more likely that those things will appear in your life. It seems that from the beginning of time to present day, man has known that getting things down — whether it be paint on rock or words on a sheet of paper — is the way to get those things for real.

That's why the people who first developed agriculture in Mesopotamia created images and statues of fertility gods. They knew that making actual images of fertility would aid in producing real fertility — of crops, livestock and even human offspring.

Still later, an ancient Egyptian healer by the name of Hermes Trismegitres went considerably beyond the cave dwellers and Mesopotamians and developed an entire spiritual philosophy in which mind was considered to be far more powerful than matter, and that mind was more powerful than the physical body.

Hermes philosophy came to be known as Hermetic Philosophy. Under this system of thinking, a person who holds a specific image in his mind strongly enough and long enough will eventually see that thing appear in his real life.

Over in India, spiritual masters there incorporated visualization practices in the ancient art of yoga. The highest form of this art was called Tantric Yoga, which became popular around the 6th century A.D. Tantric Yoga was developed to bring more focus on mind and to turn away from focus on the physical body — in other words, freeing human beings from the dictates of disease, aging and other weaknesses of the flesh.

But eastern religions are not the only ones to employ the power of visualization. Mainstream

Western religions, such as Christianity and Judaism also embraced many forms of visualization into spiritual practice. In fact, the central act of Christianity, the eating of bread and drinking of wine is a way of visualizing directly the body and blood of Christ.

During the Christian mass, the congregation is asked to think of ordinary bread and ordinary wine as the actual body of God himself. This is simply a kind of visualization that involves the use of real objects for the purpose of visualization, rather than simply forming images in the mind.

It's interesting to point out that, as we have seen, visualization is used for both spiritual means, and to gain material goods. Ancient cave dwellers used visualization to gain meat. Early farmers used it to grow better crops. Buddhists and Christians use it to achieve higher spiritual goals.

It seems to follow naturally, then, that visualization should be used to heal the body, and to keep the body young. In primitive societies, it is the shaman or medicine man who used visualization to heal the body. These shamans worked by visualizing a journey into another dimension in which they will find the essence of the soul of their patient, find what is wrong, and create healing on the most fundamental level of life. Heal the soul and you heal the body.

Back in Egypt, the followers of Hermes believethat all healing takes place in the mind. Healers there guided their patients on mental journeys in which they pictured their illnesses as leaving their bodies, and they were also taught to picture their bodies in a state of perfect health.

Primitive and Egyptian healing strongly influenced early Greek thinkers and their development of medicine. The ancient Greek combined visualization techniques with dreaming in their attempts to influence the health of the human body. To this very day, the ruined remains of dozens of Greek dream temples can still be found scattered throughout the Greek islands and Asia Minor.

Just about all of Western and modern thought has its foundation in Greek thought. Thus, it is not surprising that by the time the 1800s rolled around, many healers began to combine aspects of Greek thought on healing, with modern science and the predominant religion of the western world, Christianity.

Christian Science was founded by Mary Baker Eddy. The basis of this movement was that all disease is a product of the human mind, and can be dealt with by manipulating the human mind. You accomplish that through deep prayer, which is another form of visualization, eventually going to the mental source of the disease and finding a cure.

Finally, in this century, modern science continued to look toward visualization and its deep connection with the state of the physical body.

For example, in 1920 the American medical scientist Edmund Jacobson performed experiments which showed that muscle movements definitely followed the lead of what was going on in the mind. Jacobson asked subjects to visualize various activities, such as running or swimming, while having them hooked up to delicate sensors which could record extremely tiny movements of muscle tissue. The result was that muscles moved in ways that indicated running while the person focused on the activity of running, or swimming while the person focused on swimming.

Also in 1920, the German doctor J.H. Schultz developed something called "autogenic training," which involved deep relaxation, autosuggestion and visualization for the treatment of diseases.

Modern Medicine and the Mind

Since then, many aspects of the minds apparent ability to heal the body have been observed and studied by the scientific medical community.

For example, doctors have long observed what they call the placebo effect. A placebo is a neutral substance or treatment which has no true action on the physical body. Yet, sometimes when a doctor gives a placebo to a patient, such as a capsule containing nothing more than sugar or water, while telling them they are receiving a powerful drug, the result is remarkable healing power. Since it is clearly not the neutral pill that is doing the healing, but the mind of the individual — who is being tricked into unleashing the deep and unlimited healing power every human being has the natural potential to bring forth.

Another example of the minds astounding ability to heal is what doctors call "spontaneous remission," in which a serious disease clears up suddenly and without explanation. Doctors believe spontaneous remission is the body's natural ability to heal itself because some unknown force has triggered the process.

This mental power can work in the opposite way as well. People who are convinced that they are sick will often become sick, even though nothing outside the body produced an apparent cause. This is the principle by which voodoo and magic spells work. If a witch places a curse on an individual, and that person is a firm believer in witchcraft, the curse will be able to take its toll on the person, not because the curse is real, but because the person's belief system has a powerful control over everything that happens to the body, as well as it's daily activities.

Anthropologists have recorded actual deaths among tribes of various primitive peoples around the world — deaths that were caused by witch doctors who invoked a "death curse" on a particular person for some reason or another. Because the tribesman's belief in the curse was so strong, they literally killed themselves by subconscious action of their own minds.

So the mind is not only powerful enough to heal the body, it can also do the opposite — shut it off completely to cause death.

This effect is observed again and again throughout modern society. For example, did you know that more heart attacks happen at 9 a.m. Monday morning than during any other hour of the week? Apparently, many men would rather die than go back to the daily grind of their work after a blissful weekend of freedom and rest. The mind is strong enough to virtually stop the heart, rather than face another 40 hours of doing something it hates.

Similarly, people who are placed in nursing homes almost always show extremely sudden and rapid declines in their general state of health. The death rate for people admitted to a nursing home is more than 10 times higher than people of similar age who are allowed to stay home with family, or who remain independent. The nursing home is seen by most as the last resort, the one, final place that they will probably never return from. This works as a kind of immediate acceptance of death — and that's just what they get.

They visualize death, and death quickly follows. Are you starting to get the idea about just how powerful the mind is?

Here in the modern western world, we have been taught since childhood that the mind and the body are two separate things, and that one has little to do with the other. Such an idea developed as a result of an over-reliance on scientific objectivism, which stresses that the emotions, beliefs and all feelings should be left out of any scientific pursuit, including medicine; and on scientific reductionism, the idea that the best way to understand things is to break them down into smaller and smaller parts.

This way of thinking was not always the dominant view of the people of the world. In fact, scientific objectivism and reductionism can all be traced to just one man — none other than the great English scientist Isaac Newton.

Newton is the person most responsible for convincing all of us that the universe is made up of individual building blocks called atoms, and that these atoms are solid, like billiard balls which are inanimate, or "dead."

Even when conceding the fact that atoms are primarily empty space, most scientists today still stick to the premise that atoms at least "act" like solid objects even though they are not.

Because of this, they say it is foolish to think of yourself as anything but a biological, material being subject at all times to the laws of classical physics (as opposed to today's new quantum physics).

To be sure, considering atoms to be the solid, inanimate building blocks of everything has made fantastic feats of modern technology possible. Newton gave us the inverse square law, calculus and a new grip on the physical sciences that has allowed us to build huge cities, explore every corner of the globe and fly to the moon. Newtonian science not only revolutionized our physical world, but profoundly influenced the psychological outlook of the human race.

Since then Newton, taking a reductionist approach to all processes and objects has been viewed as the only legitimate way to solve problems and view the world. The problem starts, however, when those individual parts come to be viewed as more important than the whole, or worse, when the whole is forgotten entirely.

One of the best examples of how a reductionist approach is getting us into a lot of trouble is the global environmental crisis. Ever since Newton declared matter "dead" and all things ultimately reducible to inanimate particles, the wholesale exploitation of nature has become possible without concern that the Earth is a whole living entity which is "alive" in a very real sense.

Whenever humans tinker with one aspect of the environment a whole set of other aspects are affected. For example, when farmers plow their fields with moldboard plows leaving open soil exposed to wind and water, the result is erosion. Soil gets washed into streams and rivers, and carries harmful pesticides and herbicides with it. Silt and farm chemicals in the water choke off life in the lakes. First the smaller animals are affected, such as insects and frogs. Fish who feed off the smaller creatures are affected once their food source has been tampered with. Still larger creatures that feed off fish are harmed when their food supply dwindles. Artificial fertilizers in water can also cause some plants, such as algae, to grow out of control, soaking up all the oxygen in the water and choking off other life forms.

So we can easily see how plowing a field which is miles away from any lake or river can have a profound effect not only on that body of water, but also on the multitude of life forms which depend on it for survival.

Having too strong of a reductionist attitude — seeing only the plowed field and not what it is connected to — allows us to cause large scale damage to the whole system.

The environment is just one broad example of how Newton's billiard ball universe, and the reductionist mentality deeply influences the way humans interact with their world. Modern medicine is another.

Modern medicine is suffering from too much reductionism. Rather than focusing on the whole body of a human being, Western medicine more readily treats the individual "part" of a human being that is ailing. Modern medicine's main methodology is to manipulate the body chemistry of people with drugs, or to repair "broken parts" surgically, as if human beings were nothing more than biological machines that can be tinkered with and maintained like automobiles.

The result is a medical system that performs near miracles on the one hand, but on the other, fails individuals and the population as a whole. Western medicine can be effective, but often cruel and shockingly impersonal. Western medicine has been lead kicking and screaming toward more holistic and preventative medicine in the past two decades, but there was a time when holistic medicine was considered a lot of simple minded, unscientific fluff. Today, maintaining positive health rather than treating diseases after they happen is becoming extremely important as modern medicine inches away from reductionism toward holism.

On a more personal level, Newtonian physics has caused all of us to think of ourselves as biological machines made up of inanimate atoms that have somehow learned to act as living creatures, even though the very substance we are made from is supposedly dead. It has also influenced us to make a greater separation between mind and body than is warranted.

For one thing, it is an easy matter to see how your body is not a solid, fixed object. You body is in a constant state of growth, death and renewal. Each cell in your body is born, multiplies and is cast off at a regular rate. You constantly take in new substances from the Earth to keep the dynamic process of your body going.

As several deep thinkers have pointed out — including Buckminster Fuller, Aldous Huxley and more recently Deepak Chopra — there is not a single cell or molecule in your body that was there just a year ago. The body you were riding around in last year is completely gone now — it has been exchanged from top to bottom with new materials from the Earth and universe.

But what always remains is you. Your body is a fluxion. It comes and goes and you are the one who pivots somewhere within that process, remaining in proximity with the process until the process ends.

The sociologist Morris Berman said:

"There is no object existing by itself; every object has a stream of consciousness, or what we have called Mind, attached to it." Not thinking of your body as a hard physical object brings up the question: Where and how does my mind "ride" along on this dynamic, fluxion thing? Thinking of your body as a verb rather than a noun does not allow you to think of your brain simply as a bucket that your mind has been dumped inside. Your brain and body are not like a hard computer with information stored inside it on bits of silicon.

Your mind or soul, or whatever you want to call it, is more like a surfer. It is surfing on a biological wave of rising and falling atoms, which, in turn, are mostly empty space and bits of energy.

The most important thing to remember about all this is that your mind is the grand controller of the entire process. And it is you who controls your mind. Theoretically, you can have control over every single cell in your body. It is you who make the commands, it is the body that follows.

The simple reason that none of us are able to take advantage of this power today is the fact that we have been programmed since childhood by our society to believe that mind and matter, or mind and body, are two separate things, and never shall they meet.

How do we overcome this? Simply by changing our belief system.

How do you do that? Well, one great way is through the process of visualization. Another is through repetition of visual images. All our lives it has been drummed into us that body and mind are separate. Now we have to reverse that programming by drumming into our minds that mind and body are intimately connected, and that mind controls body.

There is a saying: "Call a man a dog once and you insult him. Call a man a dog a thousand times and he may start barking."

If something is repeated often enough, whether that be something true or something ridiculous, the human mind finds it increasingly difficult to not accept what is being repeated a truth, and reality itself.

Advertisers certainly know this. That's why they run some of the most aggravating and insipid commercials again and again. They know that if they keep beating the drum long enough and loud enough, the message is going to be driven home and accepted by the consumer. Before the consumer knows it, she really believes that a floor wax truly will make her happier and more fulfilled, or that a new car will elevate you to a new strata of society.

Repetition of an idea is closely akin to visualization in that it involves keeping the mind focused on a thought, idea or concept for a long period of time — long enough to bring the visualizer and that which is visualized together.

This power can be used for more than selling floor wax or cars to unwary consumers, but for a much greater and more important goal — giving us all the ability to have complete control over the state of our physical bodies.

Theoretically, we can stay young, youthful and vigorous for as long as we want as long as we hold a powerful image of ourselves as being that way in our minds. Setting aside 15 to 30 minutes every day to do nothing but lie down, clear your mind, and visualize yourself as being young and full of energy will probably do more than all the DHEA money can buy to keep your body in a young, vigorous and energetic state of being.

The following is a Six Step method for practicing successful visualization for perpetual youth.

1. Body relaxation

Find a quiet time of day when you will not be disturbed by anyone or anything. That means telephones, pets, the mailman, or anything else. Find a room that is quiet and undisturbed, and ideally, which blocks out most sounds.

In order to relax successfully, you must teach your body what relaxation feels like. Most people know what muscle tension feels like, but have relatively little experience with the opposite.

One of the best methods for learning relaxation is called progressive relaxation. This involves tensing various parts of your body, holding it for a moment, and then carefully observing what it feels like to let go of that tension. Many people start by making a tight fist, holding it for a minute, then letting it go. Next, they tense the arms, hold the tension, then let it go, again being sure to pay close attention to what it feels like for the muscles to simply let go. After doing every part of the body, from toes to the scalp, the individual becomes extremely acquainted with the feeling of letting go. Once you know what it feels like, you can command your entire body to produce this response, with or without the tensing and untensing exercise.

2. Mind Deepening

When the body relaxes, the mind often follows suit. But just as often, the mind races and chatters, quickly destroying all the difficult work of body relaxing.

The best way to relax and deepen the mind is to focus your attention on your breathing and away from other thoughts. When many people first do this, they realize they are breathing in rapid, shallow breaths.

What you want to do is consciously switch from shallow, rapid breathing to slow, deep breathing. Additionally, it is best to breathe with the lower stomach, rather than from the chest.

Once the breathing is slowed and becomes deeper, it's time to start counting breaths, much in the way we described in the section on meditation above. Count each completed in and out breath as 1. Keep counting this way up to four, and then start over. After several minutes of this, both your body and mind will be in an extreme state of relaxation.

Don't worry if you are not successful with these methods right away. You'll get better with practice. Resist the urge to judge yourself if you fail to get as relaxed as you think you should be. Even getting a little relaxed is a great accomplishment for many people. The more you practice, the better you'll get.

3. Prepare for Visualization

From within your relaxed state, say to yourself: "I am now ready to form powerful mental images in my mind. My mind is clear. My body is relaxed. I can hold onto whatever image I create for as long as I want." Please remember that you do not have to repeat these words verbatim, just something similar.

4. Form your Image

Now it's time to picture yourself as you want to be. Because we are talking about youth in this book, we suggest you form an image in your mind of how you would like to look and how you would like to feel. The more detailed you make this picture and the longer you hold it in your mind, the more powerful the effect this exercise will have.

You can approach this in one or both of two different ways. You can work on individual aspects of your body, or do the whole thing once. In the first case, for example, you may want to start with your skin. If your skin is currently wrinkled or blemished in ways that are not to your liking, imagine it smoothening, and the blemishes fading away. Visualize your skin as smooth and perfect, complete with a pink glow and moist feel.

The more of the five senses — vision, taste, smell, touch and taste — you can bring into the process, the more real and the more powerful the effect will be. Don't just picture your skin as smooth and perfect, imagine what it would FEEL like to have such skin. Imagine what it would sound like to rub your hand up and down your face or arm. Would it make a rough sound or a smooth swish? Once again, the more complete your image the more powerful the effect of your visualization exercise.

After you do the skin, you may want to visualize your heart as being strong, steady and clear of obstructions, such as cholesterol or blood clots. Next you can work on your digestive system, visualizing not only a healthy stomach and intestines, but the process of comfortably eating a meal without problems of indigestion, heartburn or stomach pain.

Some people prefer to visualize the entire body in the ideal condition they want it to be. Some people form a strong internal image of a lean, muscular body, full of vibrant youth and energy. They picture the body running, swimming, or simply standing in a serene setting — a picture of perfect youthful health.

Most importantly, they make the image of this body THEIR OWN body. To be effective at using visualization, you must remember to always include yourself in the image you are projecting.

5. Merge the Image into Yourself

As a way to complete your visualization exercise, mentally merge the image of the perfect, healthy body with yourself as you currently exist. For example, imagine the body you have visualized as floating directly above you if you are lying down, or as sitting or standing directly opposite you, like a mirror image. Then imagine your idealized body image coming toward you and slipping inside your physical body like a ghost image merging with your real self.

6. Repeat Every Day

The true power of visualization comes from steady practice and week after week of repetition. Remember, the human mind is conditioned by repetition. What is repeated to the mind becomes real to the mind, and what is real to the mind generally makes up the very reality which greets us in the every day world.

We strongly urge you to practice visualization once a day, perhaps for 20 minutes to one half hour per day. Doing so will almost immediately have the effect of making your body produce more natural DHEA, out of which the rest of so many other super hormones are synthesized.

Visualization is perhaps one of the most powerful youth generating techniques ever invented during the entire history of human kind.

Worry, Anxiety, Negativity — Robbers of Youth

Do happy people live longer than unhappy people? The answer has been scientifically proven to be yes! Study after study has shown that people with positive attitudes, people who are in love with life, people who have a loving relationship with an intimate partner and people who have a lot of friends and an extended support group live an average of 18 years longer than people who live alone, and who are depressed, or who have negative and pessimistic feelings about life.

Are you the kind of person who is constantly rushing from one thing to the next? Are you always worried about your job, family, money, and health? What about feelings of guilt, worry and regret? Have lots of them. Most people do. For most of you, all this probably sounds very familiar.   This is the kind of daily stress that actually steals years from your normal lifespan, and the kind of stress that can literally kill you.

A hectic life actually changes the body chemistry, something every one should be more educated about. It's well documented that when we feel stressful emotions like worry and anxiety our body produces more of the stress hormone cortisol, which among other things, dampens the ability of the brain to think clearly. High cortisol levels in women also lead to estrogen dominance, which can cause severe headaches, painful PMS symptoms and in some cases, infertility. In men, this can cause feminine characteristics and low fertility at all ages.

Scientists say that women are more prone to this kind of thing than men primarily because women generally have higher feelings of guilt and responsibility in getting things done. In general, though, both men and women have plenty of guilt, fears, worries and anxiety to deal with.

But the truth is that we can manage these daily negative emotions like worry and low grade anxiety, and create a healthier balance in our hormonal chemistry. Doing so has the effect of increasing the level of DHEA in your body, and decreasing the amount of harmful substances especially stress hormones like cortisol.

Here are some common anxiety factors for women:

➡ I ignore my kids too much
➡ My full time job does not enable me to keep up my house.
➡ I carry more burdens than my husband; he does not worry about housework like I do.
➡ I'm so worn out at the end of the day my sex drive is nowhere. Eventually my husband will look elsewhere for real, exciting sex.
➡ I have trouble limiting by burdens because I can't say no to my kids, husband or anyone else.
➡ I have to do everything myself, or nothing gets done.
➡ I have to be nearly perfect — a supermom and a superwife, or I'll be traded in for a younger, sexier model.

Common anxiety factors in men:

➡ If I don't put in a lot of overtime, I'll be passed by for promotion, or I could lose my job.
➡ I have to work so hard to support my wife and

children, I don't have any time to spend with them.

➡ I am the one who is ultimately responsible for the house, my family and everything else.

➡ Something is bound to go wrong at any time.

➡ Money is a constant worry for me. The future is uncertain.

➡ I must be successful or I'll lose my manlyhood.

➡ I am not good looking enough for my wife/women — my wife may leave me for a richer more successful man — women are looking for men that have more money and looks than me.

Common anxieties for both sexes

➡ It seems impossible to get ahead financially.

➡ I never seem able to do enough, even though I'm working/busy all day, every day.

➡ I do not feel appreciated for everything I do.

➡ I'm worried about getting old. Every day I seem to slip a little more. My skin wrinkles. My body gets flabby. My hair gets gray/thin.

➡ I never get enough time to exercise. I have a hard time controlling my weight.

➡ My kids don't get everything they should have. I never seem to have enough time for them.

➡ What will happen to my kids? Will they get into a good college. Will they be ready to face the world on their own. Have I done enough for them?

All of these constant worries take a toll. It's important to do something about this if we are going to have a chance at staying young and not finding our way into an early grave. The good thing about all of these fears and anxieties is that they are, for the most part, under our complete control. You may find this difficult to believe at first, but the truth of the matter is, just about all fears and worries are residents of our own minds, and not the so-called "real world." Let's discuss this idea a bit further. Let's take a step back and see if we can't get a greater mental grip on all this fear, anxiety and stress that seems to be a daily part of our every day lives.

It may be a fundamental truth of our existence that the reality which greets us in the world follows the beliefs and expectations we hold in our own minds. For example, people who have negative, pessimistic attitudes about life generally find a lot to be negative and pessimistic about. People who harbor fear within themselves will find that the very things they are afraid of are constantly confronting them. On the other hand, people who are upbeat, positive and confident always seem to be surrounded by abundance and good luck. **This is no accident.**

This reminds us of a quote by the Roman statesman Marcus Aurelius: "Very little is needed to make a happy life. It is all within yourself ... In your way of thinking."

To further demonstrate this point, imagine two people — one with a fear-based personality, and another with positive expectations about life.

When the first person sees a thunderstorm looming on the horizon, he may get nervous and panicky. Images of winds, lightning and destruction will fill his mind. Maybe the person will hide in the basement, curse nature and the cruel ways of the world until the storm passes. Most likely the storm will blow over without harm. But the person with a fear-based personality will suffer regardless of the storm's effect. He will feel worse after the storm because he has just endured an hour of mental pain. It is a no-win situation. Even if the storm brought much needed rain to a drought stricken area, a person with a fear-based personality is unable to appreciate it.

On the other hand, a positive person's thoughts may run this way: "I just love thunderstorms! I love the feeling of power, the fresh, electric scent of the air ... A storm is just what we need to quell this heat ... Maybe I can drive out on a country road and get some excellent photographs of lightning ... I hope there's loud thunder ... it's like nature's version of the Fourth of July!"

A positive person will think about how the rain will make the grass green, help the crops, and ensure the apple trees will produce excellent fruit in the fall.

Mastering fear and remaining calm is a major attribute of living a longer life and being more successful in everything you do, from your job to your personal relationships with other people.

In many respects, our culture is grounded and motivated by fear. Part of the reason is that fear is an excellent catalyst for a society driven by capitalism. Fear enables people to get things done, to be at work promptly, to pay their bills and to consume at a rate that will keep them in good social standing with their neighbors.

Most people answer the cruel call of their Monday morning alarm clock and cart themselves off to another five or six days of a job they hate, fueled by fear — the fear they might wind-up homeless if they don't work; the fear society will reject them if they are not productive; the fear they might be perceived as being lazy; the fear of the old Calvinist dictum: "The devil finds use for idle hands."

Most people are law abiding citizens, not because they always want to be, but because they fear the consequences of illegal acts. Some people are tempted to cheat on their income taxes, for example, but the fear of the IRS prevents them from doing it. Certainly the IRS is one of the largest fear producing institutions in the world.

If you think about it, you can identify dozens of fears that permeate every aspect of your daily life.

A lot of us grew up with the fear of nuclear war. We fear environmental pollution, crime and bad economic times. We are afraid we will never find someone to love or that our loved one will leave us. We fear bill collectors. We fear our children will get into trouble, into drugs, or that they that won't get into a good college or get good jobs. We are afraid of what other people think of us. We are afraid we are not beautiful enough, that too much television will rot our brains, and that smoking cigarettes and eating junk food will give us cancer.

And it goes on and on.

All this fear brings terrible consequences. It makes people loony. It drives up the crime rate. The United States is the most violent industrialized nation in the world. Fear covers our lives with a subtle patina of unhappiness. It is much of the reason why the divorce rate is 50-plus percent, why racism won't go away, why we keep getting into wars and why our prisons are overflowing.

The truth about fear is that it is unjustified in almost every form in which we experience it — and that brings us to an extremely important point.

Fear is not only unjustified in our daily lives, but it is also, for the most part, an illusion. Most of us actually nurture fear in our lives, dwell upon it, and given it a validity of existence every minute of the day. Most of us do. You do it, too, without knowing it.

Those thoughts which you hold in your mind, those concepts which you persistently dwell upon, form the reality of your world. Dwelling on fear, accepting it and believing in it makes you a fear magnet. Even benign and beneficial events — such as the hypnagogic state or a thunderstorm — become agents of terror when viewed through the filter of fear.

The act of overcoming the fears has the astounding effect of making you feel more free, joyful and less fearful in your waking life.

Facing fears is practice for daily living. Learning to confront what frightens you brings strength and a sense of confidence about life. You will realize that your fears are not nearly as bad as you thought they were.

Some of you are undoubtedly saying that it makes good sense to be afraid simply because there are legitimate things to be afraid of. After all, the old Soviet Union did have bombs pointed at us! Real tornadoes kill real people all the time. Forty thousand people are mangled in car accidents every year. Second-hand smoke can give you cancer, and sleeping around can get you AIDS.

Now here is something that may help you with all these everyday fears: Think about reality in two tiers, primary reality and secondary reality.

Primary reality is that which you are at the center of this instant. If you are listening to this while sitting in a comfortable chair in your living room, surrounded by all the familiar things and collections of your life, then that is the reality you have created for yourself. If you are listening to this while you are driving your car down a busy highway, that is the reality you are creating — you, the car, the highway, the traffic, the scenery, the buildings, perhaps even the person sitting with you — are the accouterments of the universe you have chosen for yourself.

Secondary reality, on the other hand, is that which you hear about from a second-hand source. Secondary realities are those far-off countries you read about in the newspaper or see on TV. You don't experience them directly, but trust the fact that they exist based on your confidence in the media which delivers information to you.

Your trust of the various media is relative. Most of you know that you can't believe everything on TV and that newspapers sometimes get the facts wrong. You always maintain a greater or lesser degree of personal objectivity. Some people put tremendous faith in the efficacy and ability of the media to channel reality "as it is" back to themselves. Others don't trust anything they get from the media. The latter are the "show me" kind people. They reserve all judgments until they can touch something with their own hands or see it with their own eyes.

A lot of the bad and fearful news in the world comes to us via secondary sources, and thus constitutes secondary reality: famine in Africa, war in Europe and the Middle East, riots in the streets of Los Angeles. You are touched or affected by secondary reality to the amount that you let it impinge on your primary reality. **A Carl Jung quote comes to mind: "Consciousness precedes being."**

Before you can perceive secondary reality, make judgments about it, have fear of it, or anything else, it first must filter through your consciousness for interpretation — the consciousness which precedes your being.

Thus, even if secondary reality exists objectively in the ordinary way most of us think about it, those events will take some shape from your individual, unique mind.

But in the more metaphysical sense, secondary reality will be subject to the reality-building aspect of your primary consciousness. Secondary reality will have its existence or not have its existence, depending on your personal will.

Under this way of thinking, if you read about nuclear weapons in Russia, they can only hurt you if you really believe that the Russians will launch them at us. If you refuse to allow such an event within the event sphere of your primary reality, then it will never happen to you.

You don't have to buy into all of this — or any of it. But what you must buy into is the fact that you have greater control over your life and feelings than you have previously been led to believe. We urge you to give this concept further thought.

The only thing you have to loose is a lot of gray hair, and what you have to gain is enormous — 20 to 30 years of high quality, longer life full of youth, peace of mind and happiness.

Special Discussion on Time

What about time itself? No book on youth renewal can be complete without talking about something as basic and fundamental as time. Yet, most books miss the opportunity to explore this issue for this very reason — time is taken for granted as a solid given, as something you can't do anything about.

But it is time which apparently makes us age. As time goes by, aging happens. If time did not go by, aging would stop, right? This might seem ridiculous at first, because obviously, no one can stop time — or can you? The fact is, as human beings we may have much greater control over old Father Time than you know.

For example, have you ever sat through an extremely boring meeting or a dinner or some situation which you thought would never end. In these cases, it seems that time crawls along at a snails pace. The clock on the wall never seems to move when you are at the office and waiting for the end of the day on a beautiful summer day. Remember those days in school when you looked at the clock on the wall a million times, and that darned clock never seemed to move?

Now think about a time when you were having a lot of fun. A roller coaster ride seems over in just seconds. An excellent movie seems to fly by and be over before you know it. You were so focused on the pleasure of what you were doing or seeing, time was almost a non factor.

Many physicists believe this is not simply a matter of perception, but an actual slowing or speeding up of time, based on what each human being is experiencing at the moment. When we are enjoying ourselves, there almost seems to be no time at all — as if it was halted during that time of fun and fulfillment. **Perhaps time really does stop when we are feeling good.**

Most of you will have a hard time accepting this because most of us have deeply ingrained or hardened within us a pedestrian and perhaps even erroneous view of time. We are accustomed to thinking about time as something that flows from the present into the future, always in one direction. Past becomes present and present will inevitably give way to the future.

This is the classic linear conception of time. Most would say this is simply common sense. To think about time in any other way seems outlandish at best and ridiculous at worst.

But ask any scientist, especially mathematicians or physicists, and they will tell you that time is not quite as set in stone as the average person thinks. Time, in fact, is fluid and possibly even, in large part, a kind of illusion. Knowing this and understanding this will go a long way toward freeing you from the confines of your physical body.

Standard science fiction stories often involve people traveling back to earlier years or periods that directly correspond with our memory or historical records of those times. As for the future, we assume that there is only one future — the future that will spring out of our present. No one can predict the future, although we can form ideas about what it will be like based on the present, by examining trends, and so forth.

But the truth is that scientists have long known that time is not that simple and not that linear. In fact, it may be that time does not "flow" at all, like a river, but rather may take it's motion cues from the consciousness of human beings, who select and mold the events of the universe by combining elements of the past and the future in a sort of dynamic present.

Most likely, there was no single event, such as the Big Bang, when the cosmic stop-watch was clicked by the hand of God to set time in motion. It's more likely that time is a circle, rather than a straight line. Any particular point on a circle can be arbitrarily labeled a "beginning" or an "end point," but there will always be a point on either side of that beginning or end.

Time never ends. Although not entirely accurate, it may be better to say that time travels in a circle and exists at all points on that circle at one time or another — or at all points all the time.

Also, time does not have a specific direction on the circle. Concepts such as "clockwise" and "counter-clockwise" are artificial creations of the human mind. Time does not have a set rate of flow. The speed of time is most likely an illusion and dependent upon the consciousness of intelligent beings to give it meaning.

Einstein, for example, showed us that the rate of time flow is not immutable. It has been theorized and scientifically proven that time actually slows down for any physical object or person that is traveling through space. That's why astronauts traveling at near the speed of light, if that should ever become possible, will practically cease to age relative to those who are not traveling at the speed of light.

Particle physicists in laboratories have shown that some subatomic particles appear to move backwards in time, and that some particles also "come into existence" out of nothingness — in other words, they come from a state of no time and nothingness to a state of being "in" time and then move either backward or forward through time.

Physicists call particles that don't yet exist "virtual particles." They exist (or don't exist — and we confess, we don't quite get it) in a "place" where there is no time and no space — nothing, effectively. Virtual particles just "pop" into existence from nowhere. If you want to know more about that, you might want to go to your library and check out a few books on quantum physics.

Anyway, the point is, we are trying to show you something about time with all this discussion. And that something is that time is a kind of illusion. Time is not necessarily something that exists in nature independent of human beings. It is a handy "tool" we use to shape our reality and to pin the events of our daily lives upon in an arbitrary sort of way. It is not arbitrary, however, in the sense that all humanity mutually agrees upon the conventional nature of the illusion.

Humanity has not always been as obsessed with time as we are in the present day. Think about those periods of history before clocks or calenders existed. Other than having a vague impression of time based on the position of the sun, people didn't chop up their days into 24 chunks called hours, and they did not measure their lives in terms of years and months. In fact, prior to the Civil War in America, most people of the world had little idea about how old they were. No records were kept for most people, and no one thought of themselves as "old" or "middle-aged" once they reached a certain artificial hash mark, such as age 45 or 65.

Time was not as "real" in those earlier years because there were not clocks on every corner bank, in every town square, or on millions of wrists. Since time was less real, it had far less influence on the way people lived and thought about their own position in the universe.

Not only do scientists agree that time as we know it does not take the same conventional form in the greater scheme of things, but Eastern religions and philosophies have long spoken about the "eternal moment," the "transcendent oneness" which exists in a state of "no-time."

Zen Master Shunryu Suzuki said in his book Zen Mind, Beginner's Mind that we all live our lives under the illusion that we have a specific date of birth, and that there will be a specific time when we will die. Rather, he says, we all exist now in an eternal present — we were never born and we will never die — we exist like drops of water temporarily separated from a giant river, which symbolically represents the universe. We are a drop of water before we become separated from the river, and we will remain one after we rejoin the river. It's just the quality of separation, he says, that makes us feel that we are somehow different; that is, alive, dead, or whatever.

The past and future exist only in the sense that they are enfolded within the present.

That's not difficult to believe, especially if we consider that our conventional view of time is heavily dependent on physical reality based in three dimensional space. We mark the effects of time by noticing that our physical bodies seem to progress in form and capacity in a linear fashion over time. To measure time at all, we must have physical objects that interact relative to one another in a way which shows us time. The position of the sun in the sky, for example, as it relates to its height above and between the horizons of the earth is how we judge what time it is. When the sun is at its highest point, it is Noon.

But now imagine the time before there was an earth and a sun, or imagine a place in outer space so distant and isolated that no stars or objects have been distributed in that portion of the universe. How would you measure time there? With no objects to observe in juxtaposition with one another, there would be just blank space — black nothingness that would seem endless and infinite in all directions. In effect, there would be no time because time can only be measured in terms of the relativity of physical objects in three dimensional space.

So as we can see, time is a creation of the human mind to a very large extent. Do you want to stop aging? Then free yourself from the illusion of time. As our discussion has demonstrated, since time is a product of the mind, the fact that you have complete control over your mind means that you can regulate the rate at which you age by consciously willing yourself to do so.

At the very least, we think we have proved our case that having fun and enjoying life not only leads to a timeless state of existence, but reduces the stress hormones and other damaging chemicals that cause us to age faster.

We urge you to give this more thought, and to dig deeper into the concept of time. Once again, the only thing you have to lose is an earlier death. What you have to gain is a long life of youth, joy and health.

Some finals thoughts on mind over matter:

What is your body made up of anyway? Some of you might say: "Well, I've heard that the human body is about 90 percent water." And you would be right. But let's go beyond that.

Sure, your body is made up of water and various organic and inorganic molecules. Water is made up of molecules, too — H20, as you know. Our bodies are made up of molecules, which in turn are made up of smaller particles called atoms, which in turn are made up of yet smaller sub-atomic particles, including protons, neutrons, electrons, quarks and so on.

As it turns out, scientists have discovered that these smaller subatomic particles are basically made up of nothing more than light-energy combined with ... nothing! Atoms are 99.999 percent empty space! Energy, in fact, is just "acting" like solid physical matter by being in many places at one time with great speed and the help of some other factors too difficult to explain here. But suffice it to say, your body, at its most fundamental level, is made up of pure light energy.

As Einstein told us, energy in the universe can never be destroyed, only transformed.

So if your body is made up of molecules, atoms and subatomic particles — which are actually whirling bits of light mixed with nothing — that makes you and your body a pretty remarkable thing! On a fundamental level, the energy which your body has is something that can never be destroyed, only transformed to a new or different level. That's a scientific fact!

Now, keep the above in mind while you consider this: If you did not know how old you were, would you really be able to tell what your true age is? Don't be so sure!

Back before the Civil War days, most people did not know precisely how old they were. Just 150-some years ago, the general public was not as "time-obsessed" or age conscious as we are. Most people had a general idea about how old they were, but few knew — or cared — what their exact age was.

The result was that people did not expect certain life events to happen when a particular age was reached. "Manhood" was not automatically gained at age 18 or 21. People did not have a mid-life crises at age 35, or expect to die at age 72. How could they expect these things to happen if they had no idea about how old they were? A man in his fifties might guess his age at 40, or even 35 if he had no true idea about his age. Most likely, he would estimate his age based on how he felt. If he felt young, vibrant and healthy, well, he would consider himself a man in the prime of his life — and his exact age would be a non-issue.

The point is that your age is far less of a solid, quantifiable and real thing than you have been led to believe in our modern society, which is obsessed by time. In our modern world, each age comes with a label or expectancy. People in their eighties are assumed to be living on "borrowed time" because we expect people of that age to die at any time. People who reach the magic age of 65 are expected to retire, and we expect their health to begin a more rapid decline.

But if you didn't know you were 65 and you felt great and loved your job, why would you retire? You wouldn't. You would not let something as artificial as a birthday with some number attached to it affect your life.

So our experience of time is basically an illusion. It truly is. Now combine this fact with the fact that your body is made up of atoms and subatomic particles that are energy which can never be destroyed. **Are you starting to get the picture?**

If you are not, this is it in a nutshell: That old saying, "You are as young as you feel" is far more true than you ever imagined. If time is truly an illusion, as we have showed, and if the substance of your body can never be destroyed, then you can easily live years and years longer if you just accept the reality of it.

There is no reason not to. Simply make a mental note in your mind that tells you that your age is nothing more than an artificial number, and that your body is a remarkable collection of super-charged energy that is in a perpetual state of existence in the universe.

The bottom line is: Aging is literally a state of mind. Why succumb to the artificiality of numbers? Instead, judge your personal age and longevity on something other than the pages of a calender. Re-set the inner clock of your mind to accommodate a life span of 130 years. With your mind leading the way, your physical body will follow. When you reach the age of 60 or 70, mentally consider yourself to be "middle-aged" because you still have another 60 or 70 years to go. Try it and see. What have you got to lose?

NOTES

_____

_____

_____

_____

Chapter 13

Special Tips on Aging Easily

In this chapter, we are going to examine special tips on aging — the kind of facts and information you are unlikely to find in any other book devoted to the topic of aging, maintaining youth, or recovering lost youth.

Here we are going to present not only new, cutting edge and theoretical information, but also very specific information which you can truly use pertaining to specific parts of the body, from your feet to your eyes and important points in between. So let's get started!

You Need Friends

If you want to stay young, it is tough to do it alone. What you need are a few friends. That's right, there is strong scientific evidence to suggest that high levels of stress combined with lack of friends and family can significantly reduce your life span.

Scientists at the University of Goteborg in Sweden took a random sample of 50-year-old men and gave them each a physical examination and psychological evaluation. Seven years later, the researchers went back to find the men, and also looked up those who had died. What they found was that, of the men who had reported three or more recent upsetting events in their lives, 11 percent were dead. All of them identified themselves as lacking family or social support.

Of the men who had peaceful lives full of friends and family, just three percent had died.

The life events most strongly related to dying were having serious concerns about a family member, being forced to move, feelings of insecurity at work, serious financial trouble and being the target of legal action. Swedish scientists think that stress may lower resistance to disease, and that lack of caring, loving people in your life provides less psychological "will" to fight off disease and to go forward with life.

Therefore, to significantly increase your chances of living longer, take a look at your own life. Do you have a family? a close friend or friends? If you don't, perhaps now is the time to open yourself up to the possibility. Now is the time to reach out to someone — after all, your life may depend on it!

Aging and Your Eyes

Did you know that many older people have good eyesight into their 80's and beyond? Growing older does not always mean you see poorly. But age brings changes that can weaken your eyes.

There are some easy things to try when these changes happen. You might add brighter lights in more places around the house—like at work counters, stairways, and favorite reading places. This may help you see better and can sometimes prevent accidents caused by weak eyesight.

While older people have more eye problems and eye diseases than younger people, you can prevent or correct many of them by:

● Seeing your doctor regularly to check for diseases like diabetes, which could cause eye problems if not treated.

● Having a complete eye exam with an eye specialist every 1 to 2 years. Most eye diseases can be treated when they are found early. The eye doctor should enlarge (dilate) your pupils by putting drops in your eyes. This is the only way to find some eye diseases that have no early signs or symptoms. The eye doctor should test your eyesight, your glasses, and your eye muscles. You should also have a test for glaucoma.

● Taking extra care if you have diabetes or a family history of eye disease. Have an eye exam through dilated pupils every year. See an eye doctor at once if you have any loss or dimness of eyesight, eye pain, fluids coming from the eye, double vision, redness, or swelling of your eye or eyelid.

Common Eye Complaints

Presbyopia (prez-bee-OH-pee-uh) is a slow loss of ability to see close objects or small print. It is a normal process that happens over a lifetime. You may not notice any change until after the age of 40. People with presbyopia often hold reading materials at arm's length. Some get headaches or "tired eyes" while reading or doing other close work. Presbyopia is often corrected with reading glasses.

Floaters are tiny spots or specks that float across the field of vision. Most people notice them in well-lit rooms or outdoors on a bright day. Floaters often are normal, but sometimes they warn of eye problems such as retinal detachment, especially if they happen with light flashes. If you notice a sudden change in the type or number of spots or flashes, see your eye doctor.

Dry eyes happen when tear glands don't make enough tears or make poor quality tears. Dry tears can be uncomfortable, causing itching, burning, or even some loss of vision. Your eye doctor may suggest using a humidifier in the home or special eye drops ("artificial tears"). Surgery may be needed for more serious cases of dry eyes.

Tearing, or having too many tears, can come from being sensitive to light, wind, or temperature changes. Protecting your eyes (by wearing sunglasses, for instance) sometimes solves the problem. Tearing may also mean that you have a more serious problem, such as an eye infection or a blocked tear duct. Your eye doctor can treat or correct both of these conditions.

Eye Diseases and Disorders Common in Older People

● Cataracts are cloudy areas in part or all of the eye lens. The lens is usually clear and lets light through. Cataracts keep light from easily passing through the lens, and this causes loss of eyesight. Cataracts often form slowly and cause no pain, redness, or tearing in the eye. Some stay small and don't change eyesight very much. If a cataract becomes large or thick, it usually can be removed by surgery.

During surgery, the doctor takes off the clouded lens and, in most cases, puts in a clear, plastic lens. Cataract surgery is very safe. It is one of the most common surgeries done in the United States.

● Glaucoma results from too much fluid pressure inside the eye. It can lead to vision loss and blindness. The cause of glaucoma is unknown. If treated early, glaucoma often can be controlled and blindness prevented. To find glaucoma, the eye doctor will look at your eyes through dilated pupils. Treatment may be prescription eye drops, oral medications, or surgery. Most people with glaucoma have no early symptoms or pain from increased pressure.

● Retinal disorders are a leading cause of blindness in the United States. The retina is a thin lining on the back of the eye. It is made up of cells that get visual images and pass them on to the brain. Retinal disorders include age-related macular degeneration, diabetic retinopathy, and retinal detachment.

● Age-related macular degeneration. The macula is part of the eye with millions of cells that are sensitive to light. The macula makes vision possible from the center part of the eye. Over time, age-related macular degeneration can ruin sharp vision needed to see objects clearly and to do common tasks like driving and reading. In some cases, it can be treated with lasers.

● Diabetic retinopathy. This disorder can result from diabetes. It happens when small blood vessels stop feeding the retina properly. In the early stages, the blood vessels may leak fluid, which distorts sight. In the later stages, new vessels may grow and send blood into the center of the eye, causing serious vision loss. In most cases, laser treatment can prevent blindness. It is very important that people with diabetes have an eye exam through dilated pupils every year.

● Retinal detachment. This happens when the inner and outer layers of the retina become separated. With surgery or laser treatment, doctors often can reattach the retina and bring back all or part of your eyesight.

● Conjunctivitis happens when the tissue that lines the eyelids and covers the cornea becomes inflamed. It can cause itching, burning, tearing, or a feeling of something in the eye. Conjunctivitis can be caused by infection or allergies.

● Corneal diseases and conditions can cause redness, watery eyes, pain, reduced vision, or a halo effect. The cornea is the clear, dome-shaped "window" at the front of the eye. It helps to focus light that enters the eye. Disease, infection, injury, toxic agents, and other things can damage the cornea. Treatments include changing the eyeglass prescription, eye drops, or surgery.

● Corneal transplantation is used to restore eyesight when the cornea has been hurt by injury or disease. An eye surgeon replaces the scarred cornea with a healthy cornea donated from another person. Corneal transplantation is a common treatment that is safe and successful. The doctor may prescribe eyeglasses or contact lenses after surgery.

● Eyelid problems can come from different diseases or conditions. The eyelids protect the eye, distribute tears, and limit the amount of light entering the eye. Pain, itching, tearing and sensitivity to light are common eyelid symptoms. Other problems may include drooping eyelids (ptosis), blinking spasms (blepharospasm), or inflamed outer edges of the eyelids near the eyelashes (blepharitis). Eyelid problems often can be treated with medication or surgery.

● Temporal arteritis causes the arteries in the temple area of the forehead to become swollen. It can begin with a severe headache, pain when chewing, and tenderness in the temple area. It may be followed in a few weeks by sudden vision loss. Other symptoms can include shaking, weight loss, and low-grade fever. Scientists don't know the cause of temporal arteritis, but they think it may be a disorder of the immune system. Early treatment with medication can help prevent vision loss in one or both eyes.

Low Vision Aids

Many people with eyesight problems find low vision aids helpful. These are special devices that are stronger than regular eyeglasses. Low vision aids include telescopic glasses, lenses that filter light, and magnifying glasses. Also, there are some useful electronic devices that you can either hold in your hand or put directly on your reading material. People with only partial sight often make surprising improvements using these aids.

Maintaining Youthful Feet

Disease, years of wear and tear, ill fitting or poorly designed shoes, poor circulation to the feet, or improperly trimmed toenails cause many common foot problems.

To prevent foot problems, check your feet regularly or have them checked by a member of the family and practice good foot hygiene. Podiatrists and primary care physicians (internists and family practitioners) are qualified to treat most feet problems; sometimes the special skills of an orthopedic surgeon or dermatologist are needed.

Improving the circulation of blood to the feet can help prevent problems. Exposure to cold temperatures or water, pressure from shoes, long periods of sitting, or smoking can reduce blood flow to the feet. Even sitting with your legs crossed or wearing tight, elastic garters or socks can affect circulation. On the other hand, raising the feet, standing up and stretching, walking, and other forms of exercise promote good circulation. Gentle massage and warm foot baths can also help increase circulation to the feet.

Wearing comfortable shoes that fit well can prevent many foot ailments. Foot width may increase with age. Always have your feet measured before buying shoes. The upper part of the shoes should be made of a soft, flexible material to match the shape of your foot. Shoes made of leather can reduce the possibility of skin irritations. Soles should provide solid footing and not be slippery. Thick soles lessen pressure when walking on hard surfaces. Low heeled shoes are more comfortable, safer, and less damaging than high heeled shoes.

Problems to Watch For

● Fungal and bacterial conditions-including athlete's foot-occur because the feet are usually enclosed in a dark, damp, warm environment. These infections cause redness, blisters, peeling, and itching. If not treated promptly, an infection may become chronic and difficult to cure. To prevent these conditions, keep the feet-especially the area between the toes-clean and dry and expose the feet to air whenever possible. If you are prone to fungal infections, you may want to dust your feet daily with a fungicidal powder.

● Dry skin can cause itching and burning feet. Use mild soap sparingly and a body lotion on your legs and feet every day. The best moisturizers contain petroleum jelly or lanolin. Be cautious about adding oils to bath water since they can make the feet and bathtub very slippery.

● Corns and calluses are caused by the friction and pressure of bony areas rubbing against shoes. A podiatrist or a physician can determine the cause of this condition and can suggest treatment, which may include getting better fitting shoes or special pads. Over-the-counter medicines contain acids that destroy the tissue but do not treat the cause. These medicines can sometimes reduce the need for surgery. Treating corns or calluses yourself may be harmful, especially if you have diabetes or poor circulation.

● Warts are skin growths caused by viruses. They are sometimes painful and if untreated, may spread. Since over-the-counter preparations rarely cure warts, get professional care. A doctor can apply medicines, burn or freeze the wart off, or remove the wart surgically.

● Bunions develop when big toe joints are out of line and become swollen and tender. Bunions may be caused by poor fitting shoes that press on a deformity or an inherited weakness in the foot. If a bunion is not severe, wearing shoes cut wide at the instep and toes may provide relief. Protective pads can also cushion the painful area. Bunions can be treated by applying or injecting certain drugs, using whirlpool baths, or sometimes having surgery.

● Ingrown toenails occur when a piece of the nail breaks the skin. This is usually caused by improperly trimmed nails. Ingrown toenails are especially common in the large toes. A podiatrist or doctor can remove the part of the nail that is cutting into the skin. This will allow the area to heal. Ingrown toenails can usually be avoided by cutting the toenail straight across and level with the top of the toe.

● Hammertoe is caused by shortening the tendons that control toe movements. The toe knuckle is usually enlarged, drawing the toe back. Over time, the joint enlarges and stiffens as it rubs against shoes. Your balance may be affected. Hammertoe is treated by wearing shoes and stockings with plenty of toe room. In advanced cases, surgery may be recommended.

● Spurs are calcium growths that develop on bones of the feet. They are caused by muscle strain in the feet and are irritated by standing for long periods of time, wearing badly fitting shoes, or being overweight. Sometimes they are completely painless, but at other times the pain can be severe. Treatments for spurs include using proper foot support, heel pads, heel cups, or other recommendations by a podiatrist or surgeon.

Taking Care of Your Teeth and Mouth

A healthy smile is a bonus at any age. Too often older people-especially those who wear false teeth (or dentures)-feel they no longer need dental check-ups. If you haven't learned the basics of oral health care, it is not too late to start. And even if you have, it's a good time to review.

Preventing Tooth Decay

Tooth decay is not just a children's disease; it can happen as long as natural teeth are in the mouth.

Tooth decay is caused by bacteria that normally live in the mouth. The bacteria cling to teeth and form a sticky, colorless film called dental plaque. The bacteria in plaque live on sugars and produce decay causing acids that dissolve minerals on tooth surfaces. Tooth decay can also develop on the exposed roots of the teeth if you have gum disease or receding gums (where gums pull away from the teeth, exposing the roots).

Just as with children, fluoride is important for adult teeth. Research has shown that adding fluoride to the water supply is the best and least costly way to prevent tooth decay. In addition, using fluoride toothpastes and mouth rinses can add protection. Daily fluoride rinses can be bought at most drug stores without a prescription. If you have a problem with cavities, your dentist or dental hygienist may give you a fluoride treatment during the office visit. The dentist may prescribe a fluoride gel or mouth rinse for you to use at home.

Gum Disease

A common cause of tooth loss after age 35 is gum or periodontal disease. Both refer to the same problem. They are infections of the gum and bone that hold the teeth in place. Gum diseases are also caused by dental plaque. The bacteria in plaque causes the gums to become inflamed and bleed easily. If left untreated, the disease gets worse as pockets of infection form between the teeth and gums. This causes receding gums and loss of supporting bone. You may lose enough bone to cause your teeth to become loose and fall out.

You can prevent gum disease by removing plaque. Thoroughly brush and floss your teeth each day. Carefully check your mouth for early signs of disease such as red, swollen, or bleeding gums. See your dentist regularly every 6-12 months - or at once if these signs are present.

Cleaning Your Teeth and Gums

An important part of good oral health is knowing how to brush and floss correctly. Thorough brushing each day removes plaque. Gently brush the teeth on all sides with a soft bristle brush using a fluoride toothpaste. Circular and short back-and-forth strokes work best. Take the time to brush carefully along the gum line. Lightly brushing your tongue also helps to remove plaque and food debris and makes your mouth feel fresh.

In addition to brushing, using dental floss is necessary to keep the gums healthy. Proper flossing is important because it removes plaque and leftover food that a toothbrush cannot reach. Your dentist or dental hygienist can show you the best way to brush and floss your teeth. If brushing or flossing results in bleeding gums, pain, or irritation, see your dentist at once.

An antibacterial mouth rinse, approved for the control of plaque and swollen gums, may be prescribed by your dentist. The mouth rinse is used in addition to careful daily brushing and flossing.

Some people (with arthritis or other conditions that limit motion) may find it hard to hold a toothbrush. To overcome this, the toothbrush handle can be attached to the hand with a wide elastic band or may be enlarged by attaching it to a sponge, styrofoam ball, or similar object. People with limited shoulder movement may find brushing easier if the handle of the brush is lengthened by attaching a long piece of wood or plastic. Electric toothbrushes are helpful to many.

Other Conditions of the Mouth

Dry mouth (xerostomia) is common in many adults and may make it hard to eat, swallow, taste, and speak. The condition happens when salivary glands fail to work properly as a result of various diseases or medical treatments, such as chemotherapy or radiation therapy to the head and neck area. Dry mouth is also a side effect of more than 400 commonly used medicines, including drugs for high blood pressure, antidepressants, and antihistamines. Dry mouth can affect oral health by adding to tooth decay and infection.

Until recently, dry mouth was regarded as a normal part of aging. We now know that healthy older adults produce as much saliva as younger adults. So, if you think you have dry mouth, talk with your dentist or doctor. To relieve the dryness, drink extra water and avoid sugary snacks, beverages with caffeine, tobacco, and alcohol - all of which increase dryness in the mouth.

Cancer therapies, such as radiation to the head and neck or chemotherapy, can cause oral problems, including dry mouth, tooth decay, painful mouth sores, and cracked and peeling lips. Before starting cancer treatment, it is important to see a dentist and take care of any necessary dental work. Your dentist will also show you how to care for your teeth and mouth before, during, and after your cancer treatment to prevent or reduce the oral problems that can occur.

Mouth cancer — an Over 40 Problem

This most often occurs in people over age 40. The disease frequently goes unnoticed in its early, curable stages. This is true in part because many older people, particularly those wearing full dentures, do not visit their dentists often enough and because pain is usually not an early symptom of the disease. People who smoke cigarettes, use other tobacco products, or drink excessive amounts of alcohol are at increased risk for oral cancer.

It is important to spot oral cancer as early as possible, since treatment works best before the disease has spread. If you notice any red or white patches on the gums or tongue, sores that do not heal within 2 weeks, or if you have difficulty chewing or swallowing, be sure to see a dentist.

A head and neck exam, which should be a part of every dental check-up, will allow your dentist to detect early signs of oral cancer.

Dentures

If you wear false teeth (dentures), keep them clean and free from food that can cause stains, bad breath, and gum irritation. Once a day, brush all surfaces of the dentures with a denture care product. Remove your dentures from your mouth and place them in water or a denture cleansing liquid while you sleep. It is also helpful to rinse your mouth with a warm salt water solution in the morning, after meals, and at bedtime.

Partial dentures should be cared for in the same way as full dentures. Because bacteria tend to collect under the clasps of partial dentures, it is especially important to clean this area.

Dentures will seem awkward at first. When learning to eat with false teeth, select soft nonsticky food, cut food into small pieces, and chew slowly using both sides of the mouth. Dentures may make your mouth less sensitive to hot foods and liquids, and lower your ability to detect harmful objects such as bones. If problems in eating, talking, or simply wearing dentures continue after the first few weeks, see your dentist about making adjustments.

In time, dentures need to be replaced or readjusted because of changes that occur in tissues of your mouth. Do not try to repair dentures at home since this may damage the dentures which in turn may further hurt your mouth.

Dental Implants

Dental implants are anchors that permanently hold replacement teeth. There are several different types of implants, but the most popular are metal screws surgically placed into the jaw bones. If there isn't enough bone, a separate surgical procedure to add bone may be needed. Because bone heals slowly, treatment with implants can often take longer (4 months to 1 year or more) than bridges or dentures. If you are considering dental implants, it is important to select an experienced dentist with whom you can discuss your concerns frankly beforehand to be certain the procedure is right for you.

Professional Care

In addition to practicing good oral hygiene, it is important to have regular check-ups by the dentist whether you have natural teeth or dentures. It is also important to follow through with any special treatments that are necessary to ensure good oral health. For instance, if you have sensitive teeth caused by receding gums, your dentist may suggest using a special toothpaste for a few months. Teeth are meant to last a lifetime. By taking good care of your teeth and gums, you can protect them for years to come.

Arthritis Advice

Half of all people age 65 and older have arthritis. There are over 100 different forms of arthritis and many different symptoms and treatments. We do not know what causes most forms of arthritis. Some forms are better understood than others.

Arthritis causes pain and loss of movement. It can affect joints in any part of the body. Arthritis is usually chronic, meaning it can occur over a long period of time. The more serious forms can cause swelling, warmth, redness, and pain. The three most common kinds of arthritis in older people are osteoarthritis, rheumatoid arthritis, and gout.

Common Forms of Arthritis

Osteoarthritis (OA), at one time called degenerative joint disease, is the most common type of arthritis in older people. Symptoms can range from stiffness and mild pain that comes and goes to severe joint pain and even disability.

OA usually affects the hands and the large weight-bearing joints of the body: the knees and hips. Early in the disease, pain occurs after activity and rest brings relief; later on, pain occurs with very little movement, even during rest.

Scientists think that several factors may cause OA in different joints. OA in the hands or hips may run in families. OA in the knees is linked with being overweight. Injuries or overuse may cause OA in joints such as knees, hips, or hands.

Rheumatoid arthritis (RA) can be one of the more disabling forms of arthritis. Signs of RA often include morning stiffness, swelling in three or more joints, swelling of the same joints on both sides of the body (both hands, for example), and bumps (or nodules) under the skin most commonly found near the elbow. RA can occur at any age and affects women about three times more often than men.

Scientists don't know what causes RA but think it has something to do with a breakdown in the immune system, the body's defense against disease.

It is also likely that people who get RA have certain inherited traits (genes) that cause a disturbance in the immune system.

Gout occurs most often in older men. It affects the toes, ankles, elbows, wrists, and hands. An acute attack of gout is very painful. Swelling may cause the skin to pull tightly around the joint and make the area red or purple and very tender. Medicines can stop gout attacks, as well as prevent further attacks and damage to the joints.

Treatments

Treatments for arthritis work to reduce pain and swelling, keep joints moving safely, and avoid further damage to joints. Treatments include medicines, special exercise, use of heat or cold, weight control, and surgery.

Medicines help relieve pain and reduce swelling. Acetaminophen or ACT should be the first drug used to control pain in patients with osteoarthritis (OA). Patients with OA who don't respond to ACT and patients with RA and gout are most commonly treated with nonsteroidal anti-inflammatory drugs such as ibuprofen. People taking medicine for any form of arthritis should limit the amount of alcohol they drink.

Exercise, such as a daily walk or swim, helps keep joints moving, reduces pain, and strengthens muscles around the joints. Rest is also important for the joints affected by arthritis. Physical therapists can develop personal programs that balance exercise and rest.

Many people find that soaking in a warm bath, swimming in a heated pool, or applying heat or cold to the area around the joint helps reduce pain. Controlling or losing weight can reduce the stress on joints and can help avoid further damage.

When damage to the joints becomes disabling or when other treatments fail to reduce pain, your doctor may suggest surgery. Surgeons can repair or replace damaged joints with artificial ones. The most common operations are hip and knee replacements.

Unproven Remedies

Arthritis symptoms may go away by themselves but then come back weeks, months, or years later. This may be why many people with arthritis try quack cures or remedies that have not been proven instead of getting medical help. Some of these remedies, such as snake venom, are harmful. Others, such as copper bracelets, are harmless but also useless. The safety of many quack cures is unknown.

Here are some tipoffs that a remedy may be unproven: claims that a treatment like a lotion or cream works for all types of arthritis and other diseases too; scientific support comes from only one research study; or the label has no directions for use or warnings about side effects.

Common Warning Signs of Arthritis

- Swelling in one or more joint(s)
- Morning stiffness lasting 30 minutes or longer

- Joint pain or tenderness that is constant or that comes and goes
- Not being able to move a joint in the normal way
- Redness or warmth in a joint
- Weight loss, fever, or weakness and joint pain that can't be explained

If any one of these symptoms lasts longer than 2 weeks, see your regular doctor or a doctor who specializes in arthritis (a rheumatologist). The doctor will ask questions about the history of your symptoms and do a physical exam. The doctor may take x-rays or do lab tests before developing a treatment plan.

HIV, AIDS, and Older Adults

Everyone talks about AIDS (acquired immunodeficiency syndrome), but few talk about how AIDS affects older people. No wonder so many older adults think they are not at risk. The truth is that 11 percent of all new AIDS cases are now in people age 50 and over. And in the last few years, new AIDS cases rose faster in middle-aged and older people than in people under 40.

AIDS is a disease caused by a virus called HIV (short for human immunodeficiency virus). HIV attacks the body's immune system. When the immune system is hurt, it can no longer fight diseases the way it used to.

People with HIV seem to be healthy at first. But after several years, they begin to get sick. Often they get serious infections or cancers. When this happens, they are diagnosed with AIDS. The most common cause of death in people with AIDS is a type of pneumonia called pneumocystis carinii pneumonia or PCP.

How Do People Get AIDS?

HIV is spread when body fluids, such as semen and blood, pass from a person who has the infection to another person. For the most part, the virus is spread by sexual contact or by sharing drug needles and syringes.

In older people, sexual activity is the most common cause of HIV infection. Second is blood transfusions received before 1985. Since 1985, blood banks have been testing all blood for HIV, so there is now little danger of getting HIV from transfusions.

Otherwise, HIV is not easy to catch. It is not spread by mosquito bites, using a public telephone or restroom, being coughed or sneezed on by an infected person, or touching someone with the disease.

Is AIDS Different in Older People?

The immune system normally gets weaker with age, but this decline is faster in older AIDS patients. They usually become sick and die sooner than younger patients.

It may be harder to recognize AIDS in older people. Early symptoms of AIDS—feeling tired, confused, having a loss of appetite, and swollen glands—are like other illnesses common in older people. Health professionals may assume these are signs of minor problems.

Prevention

Medical experts predict that a cure or vaccine to prevent AIDS will not be found in the near future. So stopping HIV depends on each person's actions. You can prevent AIDS by thinking about the risk of infection before sexual contact. Use condoms if sexually involved with someone other than a mutually faithful, uninfected partner.

Treatment and Help

Treatment for AIDS usually involves medicine, such as AZT (azidothymidine). AZT does not cure AIDS but many patients use it to stay healthier longer. Other promising drugs are being tested. Doctors are also learning how to treat the diseases, like PCP, that strike people with AIDS.

People with HIV infection should stay in touch with a doctor who knows about the latest research. For help finding the name of an expert, call a local medical school's department of infectious diseases or the National AIDS Hotline (1-800-342-AIDS).

Older AIDS patients often may not have anyone to take care of them. Help is available from local groups in some cases and from the **Social Security Administration (1-800-SSA-1213).**

Minocycline – Promising Treatment for Osteoporosis

Minocycline, an antibiotic related to tetracycline, has been shown to increase bone mineral density, improve bone strength and formation, and slow bone resorption in old laboratory animals with surgically-induced menopause. As a result of these promising effects, the National Institutes of Health (NIH) is funding a clinical trial of the drug in women to begin in January.

Lack of estrogen in postmenopausal women leads to decreased bone formation and more bone resorption, resulting in a net loss of bone, say NIA scientists

Results in animals suggest that an inexpensive antibiotic, minocycline, may not only prevent bone loss, but may increase bone mineral density beyond that of premenopausal bone mineral density. The next step would be to test the drug in humans.

Researchers studied five groups of old female rats. They removed the ovaries to induce a postmenopausal state in four groups. The control group retained their ovaries and received no medication or hormone therapy. Of the 4 "menopausal" groups, 1 received 10 mg of minocycline daily, 1 group received 24 ug of estrogen daily, 1 group received 10 mg of minocycline and 24 mg of estrogen daily, and the control group did not receive medication or hormone. The treatment phase of the study lasted for 8 weeks.

After the treatment was completed, researchers measured bone mineral density of the femur, or thigh bone, using dual energy X-ray absorptiometry, a sophisticated bone scan. The femur is made of a hard cortical bone on the outside, spongy trabecular bone inside, with an inner cavity of bone marrow. The trabecular bone (the name means "little beam") gives the bone its strength. There is more trabecular bone toward both ends of the femur, near the knee and hip joints. By measuring both total bone mineral density in the femur and specifically in the knee and hip joint regions, scientists can determine if the bone is weak or strong, thereby predicting fracture risk.

The control group of rats without ovaries lost 14 percent of their total femoral bone mineral density, 10 percent close to the hip joint, and 19 percent close to the knee joint compared to the control group with ovaries. Rats treated with minocycline maintained bone mineral density levels similar to the group of rats with ovaries and significantly above levels observed in the control group without ovaries. Previous rat studies looking at the effects of estrogen also have shown an increase in bone mineral density.

Earlier studies have confirmed the benefits of taking estrogen to prevent bone loss in menopausal women. The studies also have linked estrogen to the development of endometrial cancer in some people. Minocycline has several potential advantages over estrogen in terms of its influence on bone. Not only does minocycline prevent bone resorption similar to estrogen, but also and unlike estrogen, minocycline increases bone formation and connectivity between bony trabeculae. Thus, minocycline has an additional mechanism of action and because it is not a hormone, it should not exert adverse effects on the uterine lining.

The action of minocycline on bone formation and resorption is unique compared to estrogen and bisphosphonate, a commonly prescribed medication to treat osteoporosis, researchers said. Estrogen and bisphosphonate prevent the resorption of bone. Minocycline is very inexpensive, it accumulates in the bone, and it causes the synthesis of strong, hard bone. But scientists do not understand fully how minocycline works, so they are beginning studies to find the answers.

Meanwhile, researchers at Johns Hopkins University and the NIA are launching a 1-year clinical trial at the General Clinical Research Center at the Johns Hopkins Bayview Medical Center in Baltimore to study the effects of minocycline in postmenopausal women with osteoporosis.

Osteoporosis is a major public health threat for 25 million Americans, 80 percent of whom are women. In the United States, 7 to 8 million individuals already have the disease and 17 million more have low bone mass, placing them at increased risk for osteoporosis.

Osteoporosis is responsible for 1.5 million fractures annually, including more than 300,000 hip fractures, 500,000 vertebral fractures, 200,000 wrist fractures, and more than 300,000 fractures at other sites.

■ **Youth Within**

Moreover, individuals suffering hip fractures have a 5 to 20 percent greater risk of dying within the first year following that injury than others in their age group. The estimated national direct costs for osteoporosis and associated fractures is $10 billion-$27 million each day-and the cost is rising. Prevention is the best hope for diminishing the personal and financial losses associated with osteoporosis.

Calcium, Magnesium, and Boron — and What They Can Do For You

You have often heard the old saying: "Sticks and stones may break my bones ...", but have you ever realized what other dangers exist to your bones? How about deficiencies in magnesium, calcium, manganese, and boron?

Consider the following facts. Deficiency in manganese is found in the diets of 50 percent of all Americans, while 68 percent are not getting enough calcium. (International Conference on Human Nutrition, 1995) With back and joint problems affecting greater segments of the population, it would be helpful to know some basic facts. According to the United States Food and Drug Administration, calcium is essential to strong bones. Manganese is an essential ingredient in spinal discs, and researchers say that supplementation with manganese chelate enhanced production of disc material in degenerative disc disease.

Approximately 75 percent of the United States population is deficient in magnesium. Recent reports show magnesium to be beneficial in migraine headaches, depression, and chronic fatigue syndrome. (Properly produced magnesium chelate has reduced PMS symptoms. In general, magnesium helps in comfort and relaxation.)

You have also heard the old saying: "You are what your eat". It now appears that a more correct version of that saying should be: "You are what you absorb". A mineral that is not absorbed cannot get into the bones to strengthen them. The amount absorbed is more important than the quantity consumed.

In the case of calcium, there is widespread use of inorganic forms of calcium for supplementation, such as oyster shells. Yet by properly combining [chelating] calcium with an amino acid [a component of protein] to create an organic chelate, 57 percent more replacement calcium was delivered to the bones than with inorganic calcium.

Chelated minerals provide 3 to 10 times greater absorption than the non-chelated ones, and are thus well worth the small additional cost. Another example is magnesium, which is absorbed 87 percent when properly chelated, but only absorbed 16 percent when taken in an inorganic non-chelated form.

The mineral boron may retard bone loss. Since osteoporosis is occurring in larger numbers of the population, this is important news. Bones have osteoclasts that break down old or damaged bone cells, while the osteoblasts work to replace the lost bone. Osteoporosis occurs when the osteoblasts can not replace lost bone tissue as fast as the osteoclasts break it down. Osteoclasts deplete bone at a faster rate after menopause, leaving women at a greater risk of bone degradation. Boron appears to have a moderating effect on this process.

The Youth Power of Exercise

Ray was 58 years old. At his 40-year high school reunion, he was shocked to find out that about half of the young men who had played with him on his high school football squad some 40 years ago were dead. Most had died from degenerative diseases, such as heart disease and cancer.

In light of the fact that 50 percent of his high school classmates were already dead, Ray felt lucky to be alive. He also felt lucky because he was no picture of health himself. He was about 40 pounds overweight. He had high blood pressure and smoked a pack of cigarettes per day. He drank more than he should, never exercised, and generally had a diet that consisted of meat and fried foods.

He had been one of the lucky ones. Most people who maintain such a lifestyle can't hope to live far beyond their sixties, and many die earlier. Ray knew he was but two years away from 60, and that his chances of seeing 70 weren't so hot.

But Ray had a lot to live for. Three great children and a wife who still adored him after 29 years of marriage. He still liked his job, found it challenging, although stressful, and he also wanted to travel after retirement. Ray decided to make some changes. He was determined to give up smoking and start up an exercise program. Back in high school, Ray had been a distance runner on the track team. Although he won few races, he always remembered how much he loved running — just running — feeling good as he breathed fresh air and watched the countryside go by.

At age 58 and hefting around an extra 40 pounds, there was no way he could "run," much less jog, not even across his back yard without gasping and breaking into a sweat. But Ray didn't let that get him down. He knew that 40 years of inactivity and cigarettes could not be undone overnight. He set a firm mental intention to build his way up slowly, no matter how long it took.

In the first week, Ray huffed and puffed around his yard. True, it was humiliating, even shocking, how little his body could do. But Ray he had nothing to lose and everything to gain. He kept at his jogs around his yard for several weeks until he felt ready to try an entire neighborhood block.

Jogging nonstop around that first block was amazingly difficult, but equally satisfying. And already the changes had begun. Ray had dropped eight pounds in three weeks. He felt more clear-headed and energetic. He found less need of the stimulation of cigarettes and coffee. One success built upon another.

After four months, Ray had worked his slow jog up to a mile a day. His weight melted away from his body. He found giving up cigarettes a breeze once he began to breath more deeply and felt generally better about himself. His work became easier because his body was better at absorbing stress.

Just one month before his 60th birthday, Ray had lost the entire 40 pounds he had collected over the past four decades. The rosy color had returned to his face. He could run a 5 kilometer race like it was the length of his back yard. His appearance had changed dramatically. Although he was turning 60, it might just as well have been 40. There was no doubt, a daily program of running, eating healthy food and quitting a couple of bad habits had dissolved 20 years from Ray's body.

What can we learn from Ray's story? Plenty.

First, this case study shows us that there is no big secret to taking the years off your body. Ray didn't do anything that was particularly revolutionary. He started exercising every day, switched to a low-fat diet, and quit cigarettes. His reward for doing that was nothing less than beating a certain death sentence. Instead of having a heart attack at age 60, Ray made that milestone a new beginning for himself.

Beating the aging process can be a simple as knuckling under to common sense. Knowing what to do is not the problem. Finding the discipline to follow through is.

Most of you probably know that eating better and exercising will be good for you. But what you have to realize is that it will be better than good for you — it may literally transform your body and life into a whole new realm. It's amazing how sometimes miracles are floating all around us, and how we are just too foggy to plug into those miracles and take advantage of them.

Because there is no doubt about it, a simple exercise and healthy eating program is nothing less than a bona fide miracle waiting to happen to you.

There is more than anecdotal and circumstantial evidence that exercise can add years to your life and make you look younger. Scientists have been examining the effects of exercise on the body for decades and there is no longer any speculation about this: there is nothing better we can do for our bodies, there is no better anti-aging process than daily exercise.

It's never too late. You can be just like Ray. No matter how out of shape you are, even if you must start at the very bottom, you can begin today to turn back the hands of time. Start with five minutes a day. Work your way up to 10 minutes. Stick with it. As the days peel by, you'll soon be looking back and laughing at the old, out-of-shape, aging you. You'll looking the mirror and see a transformation take place day by day.

Whether you're 40 or 60 years old, you can exercise and improve your health. Physical activity is good for your heart, mood, and confidence. Exercising has even helped 80 and 90 year old people living in nursing homes to grow stronger and more independent.

Older people who become more active—including those with medical problems—may feel better and have more energy than ever before.

Why Should I Exercise?

Staying physically active is key to good health well into later years. Yet only about 1 in 4 older adults exercises regularly. Many older people think they are too old or too frail to exercise.

Nothing could be further from the truth. Physical activity of any kind—from heavy-duty exercises such as jogging or bicycling to easier efforts like walking—is good for you. Vigorous exercise can help strengthen your heart and lungs. Taking a brisk walk regularly can help lower your risk of health problems like heart disease or depression. Climbing stairs, calisthenics, or housework can increase your strength, stamina, and self-confidence. Weight-lifting or strength training is a good way to stop muscle loss and slow down bone loss. Your daily activities will become easier as you feel better.

Researchers now know that:

● Regular, active exercise such as swimming and running, raises your heart rate and may greatly reduce stiffening of the arteries. Stiff arteries are a major cause of high blood pressure, which can lead to heart disease and stroke.

● People who are physically active are less likely to develop adult onset diabetes, or they can control it better if they do have it. Exercise increases the body's ability to control the blood glucose level.

● Regular activity, such as walking or gardening, may lower the risk of severe intestinal bleeding in later life by almost half.

● Strength training, like lifting weights or exercising against resistance, can make bones stronger, improve balance, and increase muscle strength and mass. This can prevent or slow bone-weakening osteoporosis, and may lower the risk of falls, which can cause hip fractures or other injures.

● Strength training can lessen arthritis pain. It doesn't cure arthritis, but stronger muscles may ease the strain and therefore the pain.

● Light exercise may be good for your mental health. A group of healthy, older adults said they felt less anxious or stressful after exercising for one year.

What Kind of Exercise Should You Do?

Physical activity and exercise programs should meet your needs and skills. The amount and type of exercise depends on what you want to do. Different exercises do different things: some may slow bone loss, others may reduce the risk of falls, still others may improve the fitness of your heart and lungs. Some may do all three.

You can exercise at home alone, with a buddy, or as part of a group. Talk to your doctor before you begin, especially if you are over 60 or have a medical problem. Move at your own speed, and don't try to take on too much at first. A class can be a good idea if you haven't exercised for a long time or are just beginning. A qualified teacher will make sure you are doing the exercise in the right way.

It may take a little effort to make exercise a regular part of your life. Once you start, try to stick

with it. If you stop exercising, after awhile, the benefits disappear.

One good way to stay active is to make physical activity part of every day. Thirty minutes of moderate activity each day is a good goal. You don't have to exercise for 30 minutes all at once. Short bursts of activity, like taking the stairs instead of the elevator, or walking instead of driving, can add up to 30 minutes of exercise a day. Raking leaves, playing actively with children, gardening, and even doing household chores can all be done in a way that can count toward your daily total.

It's a good idea to include some stretching, strength training, and aerobic or endurance exercise in your exercise plan. People who are weak or frail, and may risk falling, should start slowly. Begin with stretching and strength training; add aerobics later. Aerobics are safer and easier once you feel balanced and your muscles are stronger.

Stretching—improves flexibility, eases movement, and lowers the risk of injury and muscle strain. Stretching increases blood flow and gets your body ready for exercise. A warm-up and cool-down period of 5 to 15 minutes should be done slowly and carefully before and after all types of exercise. Stretching can help loosen muscles in the arms, shoulders, back, chest, stomach, buttocks, thighs, and calves. It's also very relaxing.

Strength training (also called resistance training or weight-lifting)—builds muscle and bone, both of which decline with age. Strengthening exercises for the upper and lower body can be done by lifting weights or working out with machines or an elastic band. It is very important to have an expert teach you how to work with weights. Without help, you can get hurt. With help, older adults can work their way up to many of the same weight-lifting routines as younger adults. Once you know what to do, simple strength training exercises can be done at home. For beginners, household items, such as soup cans or milk jugs filled with water or sand, can be used as weights.

Strength training activities do not have to take a lot of time; 30 to 40 minutes at least two or three times each week is all that's needed. Try not to exercise the same muscles two days in a row.

Sample Strength Training Plan

(Always check with your doctor first. Work with a qualified teacher to make sure you are doing the exercise right.)

1) Start with a weight you can lift without too much effort five times.

2) When you can easily do that, lift it five times, rest a few minutes, then do it again. (This is two sets.)

3) Increase to three sets.

4) When you can easily do that, lift the weight 10 times in each set.

5) When you can easily do that, lift the weight 15 times in each set.

6) Once that's easy, slowly increase the weight.

Aerobic exercises (also called endurance exercises)—strengthen the heart and improve overall fitness by increasing the body's ability to use oxygen. Swimming, walking, and dancing are "low-impact" aerobic activities. They avoid the muscle and joint pounding of more "high-impact" exercises like jogging and jumping rope.

Aerobic exercises raise the number of heart beats each minute (heart rate). It's best to get your heart rate to a certain point and keep it there for 20 minutes or more. If you have not exercised in awhile, start slowly. As you get stronger, you can try to increase your heart rate. Aerobics should be done for 20 to 40 minutes at least three times each week.

How To Measure Your Heart Rate

Your heart rate tells how many times your heart beats each minute. The maximum heart rate is the fastest your heart can beat. Exercise above 75% of that rate is too much for most people.

Helpful Hints

- Choose activities that you like.
- Make small changes so that physical activity becomes a part of each day.
- Stop and check with your doctor right away if you develop sudden pain, shortness of breath, or feel ill.
- Exercise with a group, with a buddy, or alone. Pick what's easiest and most fun.

● Be realistic about what you can do.

Local gyms, universities, or hospitals can help you find a teacher or program that works for you. You can also check with local churches or synagogues, senior and civic centers, parks, recreation associations, YMCAs, YWCAs, and even local shopping malls for exercise, wellness, or walking programs. Many community centers also offer programs for older people who may be worried about special health problems like heart disease or falling. Your local library may carry books or tapes about exercise and aging.

Prostate Cancer May Be Predicted 10 Years Before Diagnosis with Repeated Measures of Free to Total PSA

Repeated measures of the ratio of free to total prostate specific antigen (PSA) in a man's blood can predict a diagnosis of prostate cancer up to six years earlier than current prediction methods.

PSA, an enzyme produced by the prostate gland, is found in high concentration in semen where it acts to liquefy the seminal fluid after ejaculation so that sperm can swim freely. Some PSA leaks into the blood stream from prostatic cells, more so when the prostate enlarges. Part of the PSA binds to alpha-1 antichymotrypsin (ACT), a protein that prevents PSA from destroying cells by deactivating enzymatic function. Free PSA (the unbound form of PSA) is active in the semen, and becomes inactive when it spills into the blood. Free and bound PSA make up total PSA in serum.

Men whose total PSA levels are high may have prostate cancer or benign prostatic hypertrophy (BPH), an enlarged prostate gland. Earlier studies have found that the rate of increase in total PSA levels over several years is one of the best indicators of whether prostate cancer is present.

Currently, most physicians test for total PSA only, which, when measured repeatedly over time, can predict prostate cancer up to four years before clinical diagnosis. Another study shows that measuring the ratio of free to total PSA repeatedly over time may lead to a prediction of prostate cancer up to 10 years before clinical diagnosis of prostate cancer.

The NIA and Hopkins team measured free and total PSA levels on stored, frozen sera from 26 men with no history of prostate disease (control), 29 men with BPH, and 23 men with prostate cancer. All men in this study are participants in the BLSA, a longitudinal study of aging established in 1958.

They return for follow-up visits every 2 years when they undergo a battery of tests including collection of blood samples. Four years before diagnosis, total PSA was significantly greater for men who developed prostate cancer (5.0ng/ml/0.9) compared to men with BPH (2.8ng/ml/0.3) and controls (0.8 ng/ml/0.1.) Free PSA levels were similar among groups at four years before diagnosis. However, the ratio of free to total PSA continuously decreased among cancer cases over the decade before prostate cancer diagnosis. At a time when total and free PSA levels were similar among groups (8 years before diagnosis), the ratio of free to total PSA was significantly lower for cancer cases (0.13/0.01) compared to BPH (0.17/0.01) and control cases (0.21/0.02). The values that most accurately detected prostate cancer were free to total PSA ratio of /0.12 when total PSA was between 4.0 - 10.0ng/ml.

The majority of men who have elevated PSA levels and have further diagnostic tests, such as prostate biopsies, do not have prostate cancer, researchers say. This study shows that the ratio of free to total PSA may be useful in helping the physician to predict whether prostate cancer is-or is not-developing.

The American Cancer Society, the American Urological Society, and the American College of Radiology recommend that men have a PSA test and digital rectal exam annually, beginning at age 50. African American men and those with a family history of prostate cancer should have the same tests beginning at age 40. In 1996, an estimated 317,100 new cases of prostate cancer were diagnosed, and prostate cancer was responsible for an estimated 41,400 deaths. Prostate cancer rates are 37 percent higher for black men than white men. Between 1980 and 1990 prostate cancer incidence rates increased 65 percent, largely due to improved detection.

Skin Care and Aging

Americans spend billions of dollars each year on "wrinkle" creams, bleaching products to lighten age spots, and skin lotions to keep skin looking smooth and healthy. But the simplest and cheapest way to keep your skin healthier and younger looking is to stay out of the sun.

Sunlight is a major cause of skin changes we think of as aging—changes like wrinkling, looseness, leathery-dryness, blotchiness, various growths, yellowing, or pebbly texture. Still, one-third of all adults sunbathe even though they know that sunlight can hurt their skin.

Your skin does change with age—for example, you sweat less and your skin can take longer to heal. You can delay these changes by staying out of the sun.

Sun Damage

Over time, the sun's ultraviolet (UV) light hurts the fibers in the skin called elastin. The breakdown of these fibers causes the skin to sag, stretch, and lose its ability to snap back after stretching. The skin also bruises and tears more easily and takes longer to heal. So while sun damage may not show when you're young, it will later in life.

Nothing can completely undo sun damage, although the skin can sometimes repair itself. So, it's never too late to begin protecting yourself from the sun.

Smoking

People who smoke tend to have more wrinkles than nonsmokers of the same age, complexion, and history of sun exposure. The reason for this difference is unclear. It may be because smoking interferes with normal blood flow in the skin.

Skin Cancer

Sun damage also causes skin cancer. The chance of developing skin cancer increases as people age, especially for those who live in sunny areas of the country. There are three types of common skin cancers:

● **Basal cell carcinomas** are the most common. They almost never spread to other vital organs, but should be removed since they will get bigger and can affect areas that are nearby.

● **Squamous cell carcinomas** are less common but are potentially more harmful because they can grow quickly and spread to other organs.

● **Malignant melanomas** are the most dangerous of all the skin cancers because they may spread to other organs and when they do, they are often fatal.

Finding any cancer early and treating it quickly is important, especially in the case of melanoma. The best defense against skin cancer is paying attention to the warning signs. If there is a sudden change in the look of a mole or a new spot, see a doctor. Look for differences in color, size, shape, or surface quality (scaliness, oozing, crusting, or bleeding). Have a doctor check any dark colored spots.

Dry Skin and Itching

Dry skin is common in later life. About 85 percent of older people develop "winter itch," because overheated indoor air is dry. The loss of sweat and oil glands as we age may also worsen dry skin. Anything that further dries the skin (such as overuse of soaps, antiperspirants, perfumes, or hot baths) will make the problem worse.

Dry skin itches because it is irritated easily. If your skin is very dry and itchy, see a doctor because this condition can affect your sleep, cause irritability, or be a symptom of a disease. For example, diabetes and kidney disease can cause itching. Some medicines make the itchiness worse.

Maintaining Healthy Skin

The best way to keep skin healthy is to avoid sun exposure beginning early in life. Here are some other tips:

● Do not sunbathe or visit tanning parlors and try to stay out of the sun between 10 a.m. and 3 p.m.

● If you are in the sun between 10 a.m. and 3 p.m. always wear protective clothing—such as a hat, long-sleeved shirt, and sunglasses.

● Put on sunscreen lotion before going out in the sun to help protect your skin from UV light. Remember to reapply the lotion as needed. Always use products that are SPF (sun protection factor) 15 or higher.

● Check your skin often for signs of skin cancer. If there are changes that worry you, call the doctor right away. The American Academy of Dermatology suggests that older, fair-skinned people have a yearly skin check by a doctor as part of a regular physical check-up.

● Relieve dry skin problems by using a humidifier at home, bathing with soap less often, and using a moisturizing lotion. If this doesn't work, see your doctor.

Sexuality in Later Life

Most older people want and are able to enjoy an active, satisfying sex life. Regular sexual activity helps maintain sexual ability. However, over time everyone may notice a slowing of response. This is part of the normal aging process.

Women may notice changes in the shape and flexibility of the vagina. These changes may not cause a serious loss in the ability to enjoy sex. Most women will have a decrease in vaginal lubrication that affects sexual pleasure. A pharmacist can suggest over the counter vaginal lubricants.

Men often notice more distinct changes. It may take longer to get an erection or the erection may not be as firm or as large as in earlier years. The feeling that an ejaculation is about to happen may be shorter. The loss of erection after orgasm may be more rapid or it may take longer before an erection is again possible. Some men may find they need more manual stimulation.

As men get older, impotence seems to increase, especially in men with heart disease, hypertension, and diabetes. Impotence is the loss of ability to achieve and maintain an erection hard enough for sexual intercourse. Talk to your doctor. For many men impotence can be managed and perhaps even reversed.

Although illness or disability can affect sexuality, even the most serious conditions shouldn't stop you from having a satisfying sex life.

Many people who have had a heart attack are afraid that having sex will cause another attack. The risk of this is very low. Follow your doctor's advice. Most people can start having sex again 12 to 16 weeks after an attack.

Most men with diabetes do not have problems, but it is one of the few illnesses that can cause impotence. In most cases medical treatment can help.

Sexual function is rarely damaged by a stroke and it is unlikely that sexual exertion will cause another stroke. Using different positions or medical devices can help make up for any weakness or paralysis.

Joint pain due to arthritis can limit sexual activity. Surgery and drugs may relieve this pain. In some cases drugs can decrease sexual desire. Exercise, rest, warm baths, and changing the position or timing of sexual activity can be helpful.

What about surgery? Most people worry about having any kind of surgery—it is especially troubling when the sex organs are involved. The good news is that most people do return to the kind of sex life they enjoyed before having surgery.

Hysterectomy is the surgical removal of the womb. Performed correctly, a hysterectomy does not hurt sexual functioning. If a hysterectomy seems to take away from your ability to enjoy sex, a counselor can be helpful. Men who feel their partners are "less feminine" after a hysterectomy can also be helped by counseling.

Mastectomy is the surgical removal of all or part of a woman's breast. Although her body is as capable of sexual response as ever, a woman may lose her sexual desire or her sense of being desired. Sometimes it is useful to talk with other women who have had a mastectomy. Programs like the American Cancer Society's (ACS) "Reach to Recovery" can be helpful for both women and men. Check your phone book for the local ACS listing.

Prostatectomy is the surgical removal of all or part of the prostate. Sometimes a prostatectomy needs to be done because of an enlarged prostate. This procedure rarely causes impotence. If a radical prostatectomy (removal of prostate gland) is needed, new surgical techniques can save the nerves going to the penis and an erection may still be possible. If your sexuality is important to you, talk to your doctor before surgery to make sure you will be able to lead a fully satisfying sex life.

Other Sexual Issues

Too much alcohol can reduce potency in men and delay orgasm in women. Also, antidepressants, tranquilizers, and certain high blood pressure drugs can cause impotence. Some drugs can make it difficult for men to ejaculate. Some drugs reduce a woman's sexual desire. Check with your doctor. She or he can often prescribe a drug without this side effect.

Now let's talk about a sensitive, almost taboo topic: masturbation. This sexual activity can help unmarried, widowed, or divorced people and those whose partners are ill or away. Masturbation is safe, and most people agree it is normal and "okay" to masturbate. If you feel your particular religious beliefs rule out masturbation in your own life, then that is between you and your God, and nobody's business but your own. Still, for those who want to masturbate, they should have no qualms about doing so on medical or psychological grounds.

We've talked about AIDS earlier, but this important topic bears some repeating. Anyone who is sexually active can be at risk for being infected with HIV, the virus that causes AIDS. Having safe sex is important for people at every age. Talk with your doctor about ways to protect yourself from AIDS and other sexually transmitted diseases. You are never too old to be at risk.

Emotional Concerns

Sexuality is often a delicate balance of emotional and physical issues. How we feel may affect what we are able to do. For example, men may fear impotence will become a more frequent problem as they age. But, if you are too worried about impotence, you can create enough stress to cause it. As a woman ages, she may become more anxious about her appearance. This emphasis on youthful physical beauty can interfere with a woman's ability to enjoy sex.

Older couples may have the same problems that affect people of any age. But they may also have the added concerns of age, retirement and other lifestyle changes, and illness. These problems can cause sexual difficulties. Talk openly with your doctor or see a therapist. These health professionals can often help.

Old Age and Vaccinations?

Shots, or immunizations, are not just for infants and children. Adults also need to be vaccinated from time to time to be protected against serious infectious diseases. In fact, some shots are more important for adults than for children. Every year, thousands of older people die needlessly.

The Public Health Service strongly encourages older adults to be immunized against influenza, pneumococcal disease (especially pneumonia), tetanus, and diphtheria.

Influenza

Usually called the flu, influenza is a highly contagious disease that causes a variety of symptoms, including fever, aches and pains, sore throat, runny nose, and chills. When older people get the flu, they are more likely to get pneumonia, lose water (dehydration), or lose weight.

A new flu vaccine is made each year because the influenza virus tends to change each flu season. For this reason, it is necessary to get a yearly flu shot. To give your body time to build the proper defense, it is important to get a flu shot by mid-November, before the flu season usually starts. Although side effects from flu shots are slight for most people, there may be a brief, low-grade fever and some minor aches and pains. According to the Centers for Disease Control and Prevention, recent flu vaccines have not caused serious side effects.

In addition to the flu shot, two anti-viral drugs— amantadine and rimantadine—can prevent or lessen infection by certain flu strains. These drugs can be used by people who never had the flu vaccine or as extra protection by those who have been immunized. They can be taken soon after the early signs of flu are felt. While they don't actually prevent infection, they can reduce fever and other flu symptoms.

Pneumococcal Disease

Pneumococcal bacteria can cause a number of infections, including those affecting the lungs (pneumonia), the blood (bacteremia), or the covering of the brain (meningitis). Older people are two to three times more likely than younger people to suffer from pneumococcal disease. It can be much more severe in older adults.

Tetanus and Diphtheria

Most people have been immunized against tetanus (sometimes called lockjaw) and diphtheria (a bacterial disease affecting the throat and windpipe). A booster shot is needed every 10 years to keep you protected from these rare but dangerous illnesses. During everyday activities (such as gardening or outside recreation), the tetanus bacteria can enter a break in the skin and cause infection. It is important to have a booster shot if you have a severe cut or puncture wound.

In most cases, the tetanus shot also includes the diphtheria vaccine. The immunity for diphtheria also lasts 10 years. The side effects of this shot are minor (soreness and a slight fever). The Centers for Disease Control and Prevention suggests the use of mid-decade birthdays as regular dates to review adult immunizations.

Other Immunizations

The Public Health Service also recommends certain people at risk be vaccinated against measles, mumps, rubella, and hepatitis B. Adults at risk include those who work on college campuses, at vocational training centers, and in the health care field. Ask your doctor or local health department if you need to have these shots.

If you are planning to travel abroad, check with your doctor or local health department about shots that may be required or highly recommended. Since some immunizations involve a series of shots, it is best to arrange to get them within 6 months of your trip.

Keeping a Shot Record

It is helpful to keep a personal immunization record with the types and dates of shots you have received, as well as any side effects or problems that you had. The medical record in your doctor's office should also be kept up-to-date.

Widespread use of vaccines can reduce the risk of developing a number of contagious diseases that seriously affect older people. You can protect yourself against these illnesses by including vaccinations as part of your regular health care.

Medicines: Use Them Safely

People over age 65 make up 12 percent of the American population, but they take 25 percent of all prescription drugs sold in this country. As a group, older people tend to have more long-term illnesses—such as arthritis, diabetes, high blood pressure, and heart disease—than do younger people. Because they may have a number of diseases or disabilities at the same time, it is common for older people to take many different drugs.

Drugs can be wonderful tools for the care of people of all ages. Many people over age 65 owe their lives in part to new and improved medicines and vaccines. But for older adults, drug use may have risks, especially when several medicines are used at one time.

In general, drugs act differently in older people than in younger people. This may be due to normal changes in the body that happen with age. For instance, as you get older, you lose water and lean tissue (mainly muscle) and you gain more fat tissue. This can make a difference in how long a drug stays in your body and how much of the drug your body absorbs.

The kidneys and liver are two important organs that breakdown and remove most drugs from the body. As you age, these organs may not work as well as they used to, and drugs may leave the body more slowly.

Keep in mind that "drugs" can mean both medicines prescribed by your doctor and over-the-counter (OTC) medicines that you buy without a prescription. OTC's can include vitamins and minerals, laxatives, cold medicines, and antacids. Both prescription and OTC drugs can cause serious problems. Be very careful to take them exactly the way your doctor advises. To be safe, don't mix them together or with alcohol without first talking to your doctor.

You and your family should learn about the drugs you take and their possible side effects. Remember, drugs that are strong enough to cure you can also be strong enough to hurt you if they aren't used right.

The following tips can help you avoid risks and get the best results from your medicines.

● DO take medicine in the exact amount and on the same schedule prescribed by your doctor.

● DO always ask your doctor about the right way to take any medicine before you start to use it.

● DO always tell your doctor about past problems you have had with drugs, such as rashes, indigestion, dizziness, or not feeling hungry.

● DO keep a daily record of all the drugs you take. Include prescription and OTC drugs. Note the name of each drug, the doctor who prescribed it, the amount you take, and the times of day you take it. Keep a copy in your medicine cabinet and one in your wallet or pocketbook.

● DO review your drug record with the doctor at every visit and whenever your doctor prescribes new medicine. Your doctor often gets new information about drugs that might be important to you.

● DO make sure you can read and understand the drug name and the directions on the container. If the label is hard to read, ask your pharmacist to use large type.

● DO check the expiration dates on your medicine bottles. Throw the medicine away if it has passed this date.

● DO call your doctor right away if you have any problems with your medicines.

There are also some things you should remember not to do:

● DO NOT stop taking a prescription drug unless your doctor says it's okay—even if you are feeling better. If you are worried that the drug might be doing more harm than good, talk with your doctor. He or she may be able to change your medicine to another one that will work just as well.

● DO NOT take more or less than the prescribed amount of any drug.

• DO NOT mix alcohol and medicine unless your doctor says it's okay. Some drugs may not work well or may make you sick if taken with alcohol.

• DO NOT take drugs prescribed for another person or give yours to someone else.

Questions To Ask Your Doctor

Before leaving the doctor's office, ask these questions:

1) What is the name of the drug and what will it do?
2) How often should I take it?
3) How long should I take it?
4) When should I take it? As needed? Before, with, after, or between meals? At bedtime?
5) If I forget to take it, what should I do?
6) What side effects might I expect? Should I report them?
7) Is there any material about this drug that I can take with me?
8) If I don't take this drug, is there anything else that would work as well?

NOTES

_____

_____

_____

_____

Afterword:

The Promise of Renewed Youth

It's one of the most fabled quests in the history of all mankind: **the search for the Fountain of Youth.** From the very beginning of the written word in ancient Mesopotamia, tales and legends have been written about foods, potions, medicines, herbs or special waters that could stop the aging process and keep people forever young.

In 1493, on the second voyage of Columbus, a Spanish explorer by the name of Juan Ponce de Leon accompanied Columbus to the New World. Ponce de Leon heard tales from the local Indians of an island called Bimini, located somewhere north of Cuba, which reputedly possessed the fountain of youth, a spring whose waters had the power to restore youth.

Even in the 15th century, the promise of renewed youth was a powerful motivator to what were then the world's greatest explorers. The search for this Fountain of Youth led Ponce de Leon to discover Florida – where he continued his search for the miraculous source of youth until he was mortally wounded in battles with Indians. Ponce de Leon died trying to find what millions of other have searched for for thousands of years – a way to stay young, a way to never grow old.

The dramatic story of Ponce de Leon represents a fundamental drive of the human race. That drive is to not only survive as a species, but to survive as individuals, and not just as individuals – but individuals who are young, healthy, vigorous and engaged in life for as long as possible.

After thousands of years of civilization, mankind may finally be coming close to one of its fondest dreams – the true attainment of long-term youth.

As it turns out, the true Fountain of Youth is not something out there in some mysterious far off land, just waiting to be discovered by some heroic explorer.

No, the Fountain of Youth is right inside ourselves, and has been there all along! We can make this claim on three levels:

First, maintaining a youthful body, mind and lifestyle seems to be intimately connected to a few hormones which are produced naturally by our own human bodies. By monitoring the levels of those hormones and maintaining them in a balance that is appropriate for a youthful body, it may be possible to not only live to ages of 120 years and beyond, but to live those years with full physical vigor.

Second, the Fountain of Youth lies within us in the sense that it is the internal intellectual striving, studying and exploring in the realms of medical science that will unlock the secrets of nature and long lasting youth. In other words, the secret to eternal youth will eventually be produced by our own striving minds.

Third, the Fountain of Youth is within us in the sense that it is our minds that truly make us young or old. The old adage, "you're as young as you feel!" may be hackneyed and worn out, but it contains an indelible grain of truth. That truth is that the mind is truly more powerful than biology.

Through mental techniques like visualization, meditation and conscious alteration of our perceptions of the subjective flow of time, we can take control over the ravages of aging and time and be master of both.

The future of the human race looks bright. In the next 10 years, medical scientists may even have the key to stopping the aging process cold.

Every person reading this book today, for the first time in history, can say with more assurance than ever: "I will never grow old."

OTHER HEALTH AND MONEY BOOKS

The following books are offered to our preferred customers at a special price.

BOOK	PRICE
1. Health Secrets	$26.95 *POSTPAID*
2. Money Tips	$26.95 *POSTPAID*
3. The Guidebook of Insiders Tips	$14.95 *POSTPAID*
4. Proven Health Tips Encyclopedia	$17.95 *POSTPAID*
5. Foods That Heal	$19.95 *POSTPAID*
6. Healing & Prevention Secrets	$26.95 *POSTPAID*
7. Most Valuable Book Ever Published	$14.95 *POSTPAID*
8. Book of Home Remedies (hard cover)	$28.95 *POSTPAID*
9. Book of Blood Pressure & Cholesterol	$28.95 *POSTPAID*
10. Good Time Money Book	$26.95 *POSTPAID*
11. How To Have It All Money Book	$26.96 *POSTPAID*
12. Over 50 Advantage Newsletter	$ 34 1 year subs.

Please send this entire page or write down the names of the books on another sheet of paper and mail it along with your payment .

NAME OF BOOK_____PRICE_____
NAME OF BOOK_____PRICE_____
NAME OF BOOK_____PRICE_____
NAME OF BOOK_____PRICE_____

TOTAL ENCLOSED$_____

SHIP TO:
Name_____
Address_____
City_____ST_____Zip_____

MAIL TO: AMERICAN PUBLISHING CORPORATION
BOOK DISTRIBUTION CENTER
POST OFFICE BOX 15196,
MONTCLAIR, CA 91763-5196